Perspectives on Quality
in American Health Care

Perspectives on Quality
in American Health Care

Edward F.X. Hughes, M.D., M.P.H. (Editor)

McGraw-Hill Book Company
Healthcare Information Center

Perspectives on Quality in American Health Care

Library of Congress Cataloging-in-Publication Data

Perspectives on quality in American health care.

Includes index.
1. Medical care--United States--Quality control.
I. Hughes, Edward F. X. [DNLM: 1. Quality Assurance, Health Care--United States. 2. Quality of Health Care-- United States. W 84 AA1 P4]
RA399.A3P46   1988   362.1'0973   88-665

ISBN 0-07-031120-X

Published by McGraw-Hill's Healthcare Information Center
1120 Vermont Avenue, N.W., Suite 1200, Washington, DC 20005
(202)463-1700

Dedication

To R.P.M., a good friend and great leader who understands the meaning of the word <u>quality</u>.

Contents

Donald M. Berwick, M.D., is vice president for quality of care measurement at Harvard Community Health Plan and associate professor of pediatrics at the Harvard Medical School, in Boston, MA.

Jack E. Christy, J.D., is senior policy analyst at the Public Policy Institute of the American Association of Retired Persons, in Washington, DC.

Catherine F. Cleland, M.B.A. is senior advisor for quality assurance in the Office of Prepaid Health Care at the Health Care Financing Administration, in Washington, DC.

Ruth M. Covell, M.D., is associate dean and clinical professor of community medicine in the School of Medicine at the University of California - San Diego.

Emily Friedman is a Chicago-based health care writer and policy analyst who completed a Rockefeller fellowship in ethics at Dartmouth College in June, 1988, and who is a contributing editor to *Hospitals, Healthcare Forum Journal,* and McGraw-Hill's *Health Business.*

Joseph S. Gonnella, M.D., is professor of medicine, vice president, and dean at the Jefferson Medical College, in Philadelphia, PA.

Lesley B. Harris, J.D., is an associate at Lillick McHose & Charles, in San Francisco, CA.

Edward F.X. Hughes, M.D., M.P.H., is the director of the Center for Health Services and Policy Research, and professor of hospitals and health services management, and policy and environment, in the J.L. Kellogg Graduate School of Management, and professor of community health and preventive medicine in the Medical School, at Northwestern University, in Evanston, IL.

Thomas R. Hyngstrom, Ph.D., is executive director of the Crescent Counties Foundation for Medical Care, in Naperville, IL.

William A. Knaus, M.D., is director of ICU research, professor of anesthesiology, and director of the ICU unit at George Washington University, in Washington, DC.

Robert B. Keller, M.D., is associate professor of orthopaedic surgery at the University of Massachusetts Medical School, is orthopaedic study group leader of the Maine Medical Assessment Program, and has a clinical practice of orthopaedic surgery in Belfast, ME.

Barry J. London, J.D., is a partner at Lillick McHose & Charles, in San Francisco, CA.

Daniel Z. Louis is managing director of the Center for Research in Medical Education and Health Care, and research assistant professor of family medicine, at Jefferson Medical College, in Philadelphia, PA.

Christy Moynihan, Ph.D., is director of research at SysteMetrics/McGraw-Hill, in Santa Barbara, CA.

James S. Roberts, M.D., is senior vice president for research and planning at the Joint Commission on Accreditation of Healthcare Organizations, in Chicago, IL.

Andrew Webber is executive vice president of the American Medical Peer Review Association, in Washington, DC.

Karl D. Yordy is director of the division of health care services at the Institute of Medicine of the National Academy of Sciences, in Washington, DC.

First and foremost, I would like to thank the authors of the fourteen chapters of this book for tirelessly devoting their energies to writing their chapters, often within hectic professional schedules, and then rewriting them through several drafts. I would also like to thank those who proofread the drafts and offered their valuable suggestions: Blair Gifford and Martin McCarthy, Ph.D., of the Center for Health Services and Policy Research of Northwestern University, and Barbara Kremer, Ph.D., of the American Board of Medical Specialties, Evanston, IL, and Northwestern University. Blair also played a substantial role in the production of various drafts, the gathering of much of the information on the authors, and many other tasks. I am also indebted to Judith Hicks for her assistance in assembling the authors; in communicating with them on an ongoing basis; in editing, typing, and retyping a number of the chapters; and otherwise facilitating the production of this book. Thanks are also due to Phyllis Breit, Jonathan Fine, and Michelle Nesbitt for their indefatigable work in the typing of the various drafts. I would also like to thank my colleagues in the Center for Health Services and Policy Research for their forbearance and understanding when the time of the above individuals was devoted to producing the book.

A special word of thanks is due to Jim Fullerton, formerly of the McGraw-Hill Healthcare Information Center in Washington, DC, for his support in the conceptualization of the book and his understanding and patience as the true depth and breadth of the work involved in making it a reality became apparent. He was a genuine pleasure to work with. The support throughout the entire effort of Luci Koizumi, current publisher in the Healthcare Information Center, and John Christoffersson, of the McGraw-Hill Healthcare Group, is also gratefully acknowledged. Deborah Glazer, sponsoring editor, worked long hours with unending good humor to see the book through to its successful completion.

The book took almost 14 months from conceptualization to completion. That period of time witnessed its component parts being worked on in a variety of far-flung settings. I would like to thank the staff of the sales and catering department of the "Antlers at Vail" in Vail, Colorado, for the use of their copier and Ed Gilroy of "Ellington's," St. John, U.S. Virgin Islands, for the use of a phone when no other was available. Both greatly expedited the production of the book.

Above all, I would like to thank my family who for 14 months did not see as much of their husband or father as we all would have liked. But for the special dedication given earlier, the book would have been dedicated to them.

Edward F.X. Hughes

Perspectives on Quality in American Health Care

The three competing forces in the delivery of health care have long been expressed in the trichotomy of cost, quality, and access. The 1960s saw major advances both in enhancing access to care through our public programs and in our ability to measure the resulting changes in access. As a result of the growth of costs associated with that expanded access, the 1970s and 1980s saw major advances in the field of health economics. With them came greater understanding about the causes contributing to the growth in costs and the development of incrementally effective mechanisms to deal with that growth. To the general observer of our health care system, however, attention to quality has seemed to lag behind the other two.

Indeed, it is still not unusual to hear an otherwise savvy clinician or health care manager allege that quality cannot be defined or measured. Lip service has long been given to the need for quality by both the public and private sectors, but there has been a widespread perception that no one really knows very much about it or can do very much about it. Nevertheless, major advances have been made in our approaches not only to defining and measuring quality in health care but also in applying these advances in both clinical settings and public review programs. The advances alluded to in addressing costs (e.g., the implementation of DRGs and the penetration of HMOs) have brought about a new awareness of the importance of quality in the delivery of health care and a concern that quality be assured in the care delivered. As a result, there has been a major outpouring of recent legislation directed at both assessing and assuring quality in our public programs, and the mandate of Medicare's review organizations has been substantially expanded to encompass quality. In the process, quality has grown from the purview of a small group of committed researchers and clinicians to become a major focus of national health policy.

The goal of this book is to impart to health care managers and clinicians a working knowledge of many of these recent advances regarding quality in health care: to explore its definition and measurement and to provide an overview of selected instances of what is being done to assess and assure it in the public and private sectors.

To accomplish this goal, we have assembled contributions from leaders from a number of segments of our health care industry, each of whom is grappling with quality in a substantive way. They include clinicians and researchers attempting to define and measure quality; a leader in the policy community detailing advances in the public sector; front-line managers and clinicians actually assessing and enhancing quality in both the fee-for-service and managed care arenas; policy analysts both advocating for quality and attempting to design programs to assure and assess it; an educator trying to inculcate its principles and approaches in young health professionals; lawyers guiding those attempting to assess it; and a distinguished journalist observing all of the above and raising critical questions as to our society's overall effectiveness in dealing with quality. The cumulative result of what has been, and is being, accomplished in each of these areas is impressive, and the central issues being faced are critical to the future of our health care system.

We have invited the authors to address the topics from their perspectives. The result is a freshness of approach as well as a variation in style. At times, the synergy between the chapters is striking. Although the book was designed to be read from beginning to end, each chapter can be read as a stand-alone piece and in any sequence. To enhance the cohesion among chapters, there are frequent references within them to where the topic under discussion is addressed elsewhere in the book, and redundancy is kept to an absolute minimum. Different perspectives lead to disagreements, which in this book lead to lively and stimulating reading.

Like any book, there are limits to what can be included. Ideally, we would like to have seen more in the book on long term care, particularly in the area of home health care, as well as contributions from any number of distinguished researchers advancing our knowledge of quality across the country. The book is broad enough to serve as a primer for one approaching the topic of quality for the first time and yet substantive enough to serve as an update or refresher for those familiar with it. A lot of time and effort has gone into making the book comprehensible and informative for our readers. Happy reading!

Edward F.X. Hughes, M.D., M.P.H.
Evanston, Illinois
July 1988

Chapter 1

Quality Health Care:
Its Definition and Evaluation*

James S. Roberts, M.D.

The quality of the health care being delivered in this country is now under a microscope. Once considered the sole domain of health professionals, quality is now of interest to consumers, insurers, government, and business. This attention, coupled with a growing capability to collect, store, and efficiently analyze large clinical data bases, has given compelling force to those who seek greater public accountability from the health care field.

In this chapter, I will construct a framework for the definition and evaluation of the quality of health care. It is my hope that this construct will be helpful to those involved in: (1) quality assurance and assessment; (2) the analysis of practice patterns; (3) the study of clinical decision making; and (4) the analysis of clinical efficacy.

I will start by outlining my views of the purpose of health care and suggest a definition of quality which flows from this purpose. I then will discuss the various units of analysis and types of measures which can be the subject of quality evaluation and outline the types of measures which can be used. I will provide a description of the major features of an effective quality evaluation program and conclude by illustrating how this total construct can be used to evaluate quality in a variety of situations.

---

*The views expressed in this paper do not necessarily represent those of the Joint Commission on Accreditation of Healthcare Organizations.

A DEFINITION OF QUALITY

Until recently, there has been a rather schizophrenic approach to the issue of quality in health care. On the one hand, the Joint Commission on Accreditation of Healthcare Organizations, the courts, and government regulators have expected health care organizations to establish quality assurance programs to define, monitor, and improve the quality of the care they deliver. On the other hand, there has been a strong sentiment that quality could be neither defined nor measured. These competing perspectives have joined with concerns about professional liability and antitrust, among many others, to create great caution and even inertia in attempts to establish effective mechanisms for quality assurance. Recently, however, the forces of change in health care have prompted enough skepticism about the health care field's inability to define, measure, and improve quality that there is now an unstoppable demand for clarity concerning the parameters of quality health care and for the creation of effective mechanisms to evaluate and improve care.

But what is quality care? Those demanding accountability from the health care field have very different perspectives. There are those who argue that "quality" is a very individualized concept --a view captured in the phrase "quality is in the eye of the beholder." Pirzig, in his influential book, *Zen and the Art of Motorcycle Maintenance,* succinctly describes the resulting confusion:

> Quality . . . you know what it is, yet you don't know what it is. But that's self-contradictory. But some things are better than others, that is, they have more quality. But when you try to say what the quality is, apart from the things that have it, it all goes poof! There's nothing to talk about. But if you can't say what Quality is, how do you know what it is, or how do you know that it even exists? If no one knows what it is, then for all practical purposes it doesn't exist at all.[1]

Others believe that quality can be measured. Some of them translate Deming's[2] and Crosby's[3] notions from business into the health care field. They believe that quality, as Crosby suggests, should be defined as "conformance to requirements." The key then becomes the specification of the requirements.

4

When one more closely examines these two potentially polar views on quality, one is struck by the fact that they differ only if there is marked difference in the individual views of those "beholding" quality. That is, if the requirements of which Crosby speaks are generally acceptable statements of the individual views of quality, then the definitions are not polar opposites but rather are the overlapping circles of a Venn diagram.

However one chooses to define quality, it is clear in the health field that we no longer can accept a highly individualized "eye of the beholder" view. The definition and measurement of quality must be more precise. Society now demands such from an industry consuming more than one of every ten of our economy's dollars. My hope is that, as we move toward such precision, we will do so guided by active dialogue among consumers, practitioners, health care organizations, purchasers, government, and insurers. Such discussion, if constructive, will prompt needed clarification of each party's perceptions of quality and contribute to the development of a consensus on the principle characteristics of quality health care. Such a consensus will enhance the broad base of support necessary for continued improvement in the quality of care.

In order to foster such a consensus, it is important to begin the process of defining quality in health care by focusing upon the basic purpose of health care. In my view, health care exists to prevent and treat human illness. While not particularly profound, this statement is useful in helping to focus our approach on evaluating the quality of health care. A more complete rendition of this statement of purpose might be:

> The purpose of health care is to identify, in an accurate, complete, and timely manner, the health care needs (educational, preventive, restorative, and maintenance) of an individual or group and to apply the resources (human and other) necessary to meet these needs in a timely manner and as effectively as the practical state-of-the-art allows.

If one accepts this statement of purpose, one is led to a definition of quality that identifies those elements of care which are necessary to meet patient needs. I believe there are seven such interrelated elements and so suggest the following definition:

Quality health care is health care that meets the needs of individuals or groups by being *available* and *accessible* when necessary; being *appropriate* to the needs of the individual being treated; answering the reasonable expectations of those being treated (*acceptable*); being effectively coordinated across practitioners, organizations, and time (*continous*); adhering to the state-of-the-art for health care management, education, prevention, diagnosis, and treatment (*professionally competent*); and being provided in a physically safe environment (*physically safe*).

These seven elements of quality are shown in Table 1 and are discussed briefly below.

Availability and Accessibility

The "front-end" prerequisite for any health care service is that it be both available and accessible to those who need it. Few would argue that when needed health services are not available in a given community (i.e., they do not exist) or, if available, are not readily accessible, poor quality care results. Availability and accessibility may be limited by geography, individual or community financial resources, insurance coverage, the scope of a health care organizations's services, and the manner in which those services are structured and delivered. While many of these variables are beyond the control of a health care practitioner or organization, some are not. If a hospital's program for acute alcohol detoxification does not include arrangements for long-term follow up (whether directly or by effective referral), it ignores the essential fact that alcoholism is a chronic disease. Arbitrary and rigidly enforced limitations on outpatient mental health services do not reflect the prolonged nature of many mental health "crises" and may be shortsighted in their cost savings objectives. Comprehensive managed care programs in which ambulatory care services are not located within reasonable distances of the enrolled populations also are not providing high quality care.

At a more subtle level are the situations where patients could benefit from subspecialty consultation or diagnostic procedures which are not easily accessible. Is this poor quality care? I believe it is. I also acknowledge, however, that there are situations in which individuals have freely chosen a geographic place of residence; e.g.,

6

a very rural area, and, with that, a possibility that health care, which is generally readily available in more populated areas, may be more difficult to obtain. In such situations, the test of the quality of the care is whether the patient needing more specialized care is made aware of this need and is aided in seeking it.

For example, in the Joint Commission's accreditation of hospitals, we have struggled with such a situation regarding inpatient obstetrical care. The Joint Commission's standards require that anesthesia services be available within thirty minutes whenever a hospital provides obstetrical deliveries. We have surveyed a few geographically remote hospitals that have no on-site anesthesia capability but do offer obstetric care. Women in these hospitals needing emergency cesarean sections must thus be transferred to hospitals more than thirty minutes away. Some of these hospitals lacking anesthesia capacity, however, are part of highly organized regional systems of prenatal, intranatal, and postnatal care, each of which is targeted to a clearly defined population. Each of these populations appears to understand and know how to use the system properly. Statistics on deaths and complications are consistent with these systems providing very high quality care.

The Joint Commission has chosen to accredit these hospitals because: 1) their patient populations have been informed both about the limited nature of the services available in their communities and the means of obtaining emergency services, and 2) the overall clinical results have been exceptionally positive. In this case, a difficult access problem has been recognized and addressed effectively. By encompassing all phases of obstetrical care, these above systems are able to offer a narrow range of obstetrical care in the rural hospitals by enhancing transfer and referral capabilities. Such planning helps to assure availability and access to needed services.

Thus, availability and accessibility have at least five important dimensions which can be considered in evaluating quality:

- Recognition of the need for a given service;
- Physical/geographical availability of these services;
- Information to patients concerning the availability and accessibility of services they need;
- Financial accessibility to the services; and
- Transportation to reach the needed service.

Appropriateness

From the inception, in 1966, of Medicare's utilization review requirements, the concept of appropriateness has been closely linked with attempts to limit resource use and, thereby, to control costs. Judgments concerning the appropriateness of given health care services most often have focused upon the site of care (does this patient need to be hospitalized?) and duration of care (when can this patient be discharged?). Since decisions in these matters influence physician and hospital income, they have created such tension among regulators, health care professionals, hospitals, and patients that a more important question regarding appropriateness has been largely ignored; namely, are the specific services received by patients appropriate to their health care needs, regardless of the site or duration of care? This issue is now receiving more attention as data concerning practice variation surface and prompt questions about the nature of clinical decision making. This dimension of appropriateness has two components. The first concerns efficacy: does the service have any proven efficacy? In other words, does it work? The second concerns the proper application of efficacious services: is the service effective for the needs of the specific patient? Each of these components of appropriateness is addressed briefly below.

In two important papers recently commissioned by the National Leadership Commission for Health Care, Wennberg and Eddy and Billings graphically illustrate the paucity of scientific evidence available to guide health care practitioners in many of their day-to-day clinical decisions.[4,5] Practitioners often cannot know the degree of probability that a given service will help a specific patient, because the data necessary for such knowledge simply do not exist. This "clinical uncertainty" no doubt contributes much to the variation in practice which has been shown to exist between counties,[6,7] across small geographic regions,[8,9,10] among hospitals,[11] and for specific operative procedures.[12] In Chapter 8 of this book, Keller presents a methodology to reduce this variation.

Of equal importance is that element of appropriateness which relates to the proper application of the knowledge which does exist. Key questions here are: 1) will the results of a diagnostic service materially aid in establishing a patient's diagnosis or in eliminating one or more possible diagnoses; 2) will a therapeutic procedure contribute to the alleviation of a patient's symptoms; and 3) of all possible services, which has (have) the highest probability of helping this patient?

Thus, appropriateness has four key dimensions which can be considered in the evaluation of quality:

- Appropriateness of the site of care;
- Appropriateness of the duration of care;
- Avoidance of services with unproven efficacy; and
- Proper use of services which have proven efficacy.

Acceptability

Acceptability is a component of quality which is receiving more attention as health care becomes more competitive. Until recently, this element of quality was thought of as "patient satisfaction" and was often considered to be the domain of public relations departments of health care organizations. The issues studied related to patients' or their families' satisfaction with convenience (appointment availability, waiting room times), communication (clarity, openness, responsiveness), and comfort. Most often these efforts were prompted by a desire to assure a level of customer satisfaction which would foster continued use of services.

As competition is growing in local health care markets, more attention is being devoted to acceptability. There is, simultaneously, an expansion in focus to more clinically related measures and an expansion in the audiences interested in this topic. I will address these important changes, starting with the last point. As noted before, attention to patient satisfaction has traditionally been prompted by a desire to have the patient continue to use the organization in the future and to recommend it to others. The focus was the individual patient. In a highly competitive marketplace, however, survival of a health care organization depends not only upon the satisfaction of the patient, but also upon the satisfaction of the patient's employer, the payer, who must decide whether to continue to offer the health plan, preferred provider organization, etc., to employees. Thus, we are seeing health care organizations now trying to understand the health benefits manager's view of quality and reorient their efforts to satisfy this important customer.

Likewise, there is an expansion in the measures used to monitor the acceptability of care. While issues of convenience, communication, and comfort remain important, there is a growing interest in the outcomes of care. Specifically, patients are more intent on assuring that the care they anticipate receiving will produce the results they desire: What evidence is there that my pain will be relieved? Will the surgery you recommend cure my problem?

In a similar but differently targeted manner, employers increasingly want to know an organization's track record on their return of workers to full productivity after the workers receive care from that organization. Similarly, they will want to know the degree to which a health care organization's educational and treatment programs have prevented the occurrence of new health problems in their employees. Thus, current narrowly conceived notions of satisfaction will expand to meet these more sophisticated, expectation-based, measures of acceptability. Health care organizations in the future will be devoting increasing resources to the evaluation of the acceptability of the care they provide, if for no other reason than the fact that, as in most other industries, customer acceptance of a health care organization may well be the most important determinant of organizational survival.

Before summarizing the critical components of acceptability, it is important to point out that convenience, communication, and comfort (the "soft" factors) can influence the outcomes of care (the "hard" measures). Effective communication and sensitive attention to patient anxiety are not just "nice" things to do. A well informed, reasonably calm patient and family are better able to understand treatment options, make informed decisions, participate in the care being rendered, and have a realistic understanding of the projected results of care. If a health care organization wants to maximize the "hard" data of expected outcomes, it is important that they attend to "soft" matters of convenience, communication, and comfort.

Thus, the important determinants of acceptability are:

- Effective communication;
- Convenience and comfort;
- Attention to the fears and concerns of patients and their families;
- Clear understanding of patient expectations concerning the results of care; and
- Measures and communication of the differences between patient expectations and both projected and actual outcomes.

Professional Competence

The delivery of health care is a human endeavor. Though aided by technology, health care remains essentially a process of humans interacting with humans. To meet human needs effectively, health care must be provided by competent practitioners working closely with (or within) health care organizations which are governed and managed by equally competent individuals.

Health care is no easy task. It is made complex by the previously mentioned uncertainty of medical science, by the variation among patients in the physical and psychological expressions of disease, and by the frequent need for coordination of skills and services of several practitioners and organizations in the care of an individual patient. Overcoming this complicated set of challenges requires practitioners well versed in state-of-the-art medical care and well-managed organizations committed to the delivery of high-quality care.

As noted earlier, the essence of high-quality clinical performance is the timely use of effective educational, preventive, diagnostic, and therapeutic services to identify and meet patient needs. In its simplest form, the care of patients includes several sequential steps: 1) assessment, 2) problem identification/diagnosis, 3) treatment, and 4) ongoing monitoring. This process is iterative, with monitoring often prompting reassessment and subsequent modification of diagnosis and treatment. To be successful, the process requires the active participation of patients and their loved ones and, often, the coordinated efforts of several practitioners. Central to success is the proper application of the collective body of medical knowledge and individual practitioner skill to accurately identify health problems and treat them as effectively as possible.

Thus, both a collective prerequisite and an individual component determine the ability of a practitioner to help a patient. The collective component concerns our existing state of knowledge. As noted earlier, Eddy and Billings have shown that much of health care lacks a firm scientific base. New procedures are often adopted without adequate clinical trials. There is often a tendency to use accepted clinical procedures in untested ways. The competent practitioner (or team of practitioners) is challenged constantly to stay current with the evolving state of knowledge and to apply it with the interpersonal and physical skills required to achieve optimal results.

The importance of competent individual practitioners is matched by the necessity of enlightened and competent governance and management. By comparison with other segments of our economy, the effective exercise of governance and management responsibilities in health care has received little attention. Yet, society holds the governing bodies of health care organizations responsible for the quality of care provided by the organization. Managers are challenged by rapidly evolving regulatory and economic pressures which require increased organizational competitiveness. This, combined with the inherent complexity of health care, has focused more attention both on the careful selection of board members and senior managers and on the effective exercise of institutional policy making and administrative responsibilities.

For decades, the regulations of state and federal governmental agencies and the standards of private accrediting organizations have specified characteristics of organizational structure and function which are believed to be related to the delivery of high quality care. As an early component of a now active attempt to recast and improve the relevance of those standards, Steven Shortell, Ph.D., of Northwestern University, and I have developed the following list of organizational characteristics we believe are related to quality:[13]

1. Clarity of the purpose of the organization;
2. Establishment of an organizational design and corporate culture capable of achieving the stated purpose;
3. Establishment of, and committment to, high standards;
4. Competence in governance and management as evidenced by such characteristics as: the ability to look to the future and stimulate strategic movement toward it, willingness to take prudent risk, the ability to oversee and manage change effectively, the ability to learn from mistakes, the persistence in pursuing improvement, and the ability to manage conflict;
5. Competence in clinical practice;
6. Consistent emphasis on, and support for, professional growth;
7. Effective and timely coordination of management and clinical services within the organization and its practitioners and among organizations;

12

8. Assurance of the availability and accessibility of the organization's services to its patient population;

9. Consistent application of contemporary standards of good clinical practice and achievement of reasonable expectations of service effectiveness;

10. Effective monitoring of the quality of care, correction of deficiencies, and timely improvement of care consistent with advances in the state-of-the-art of health care;

11. Meeting the reasonable expectations of patients; and

12. Assurance of a physically safe environment.

This list of characteristics and those supplied by others are now being refined by an expert task force appointed by the Joint Commission to specify the major characteristics of organizational structure and function which are essential to the provision of high quality care. A central theme likely to emerge from this work is the critical importance of a top-to-bottom organizational commitment to continual improvement in the quality of care.

Continuity

The sixth element in quality health care is continuity of care --the timely flow of care among practitioners, organizations, and time. This component has taken on greater meaning as practitioners of all types have subspecialized, as health care organizations have proliferated in local communities and developed formal and informal referral patterns, and as chronic disease prevalence has increased with the aging of the population. Achieving coordination of care is dependent principally upon the timely transfer or referral of the patient and the transmission, also in a timely manner, of the information needed to effectively continue that care.

To illustrate the importance of timely information transfer, consider a hospital that has shifted much of its surgery from an inpatient to ambulatory mode. A patient requiring a herniorrhaphy in the past would have been admitted to the hospital, where the physician's admission note would have summarized for hospital personnel the patient's pertinent clinical and social information. Nursing and anesthesia practitioners could digest this information, spend time with the patient, and therein reasonably assess the objective risk of the procedure. When the procedure is performed on an ambulatory basis, however, the patient often arrives at the ambulatory facility just prior to surgery. Thus, the patient's clinical situation must be assessed more rapidly by those providing and supporting the care. This means that information that formerly was gathered over several hours (vital signs, comorbidities and their severity, the presence of allergies, lab test results, level of anxiety, anesthesia risk, and precise nature of the procedure) must be obtained and synthesized in a much shorter period. In addition, complications of the surgery, which in the past would have occurred during hospitalization, now often occur after discharge. Thus, information pertinent to the evaluation of the quality of surgical care must now also be obtained from the patient or practitioner after discharge. This is no easy task.

Appropriate information flow in this and similar situations (e.g., between a nursing home and a hospital for a patient to be admitted from the nursing home; between a home care agency and an attending physician; between a hospital-based detoxification program and a residential alcohol treatment program) requires: 1) agreement upon the general nature of that information; 2) systems to gather and collate the information from multiple sources; and 3) the time and diligence to use it appropriately in planning for the care of the patient. These important characteristics of information gathering, exchange, and use should be the subject of quality of care evaluation.

Continuity of care is also important during hospitalization. Consider the patient with an acute, complex, multiorgan disease requiring the care of several physicians. Here, subspecialization can be both a blessing and a problem. Each subspecialist embodies the potential for effective treatment of the disease processes affecting "his" organ system. The patient is not merely a collection of unrelated organ systems, however. The care given by one specialist often affects that given by others and thus must be coordinated in some way, most preferably by a physician who has primary responsibility for the patient. Such coordination is often not easily accomplished and requires each practitioner to communicate with colleagues in a timely and accurate manner and with sensitivity to the level of knowledge of those colleagues. Again, the nature and success of such coordination can, and should, be the subject of quality assurance programs.

Finally, consider the problem of continuity of care for those with chronic illness. For example, consider the care needed by an individual with progressively debilitating rheumatoid arthritis. In this situation,

14

a primary care practitioner and a rheumatologist may need to work for years with various medications to control symptoms. Later in the course of the disease, surgery may often be required and the care of physical and occupational therapists may be needed to sustain daily living activities. Concomitant with the joint disease may come other organ involvement and the parallel development of unrelated acute and chronic diseases. When considering this years-long chronology, one can appreciate the persistence needed to effectively communicate information between practitioners; and, the importance of succinctly summarizing that information so that a practitioner can quickly ascertain where the patient has been therapeutically in the past.

Physical Safety

Often considered to include only fire safety, this element of quality actually has many important dimensions. They include safe disposal of material contaminated with biological and nuclear wastes, accurate calibration and ongoing maintenance of potentially dangerous equipment, and effective planning for natural and man-made disasters. The Joint Commission on Accreditation of Healthcare Organizations has produced a series of publications providing guidance on each of these matters and their integration into a well managed plant, technology, and safety management program.[14]

EVALUATING QUALITY--WHAT IS THE UNIT OF ANALYSIS?

The next step in constructing an approach to evaluating quality of care is to consider the possible levels or components of the health care system which can be analyzed. I believe there are four possible units of analysis: the patient-individual practitioner interaction, the patient-practitioner team interaction, the health care organization, and the community. I have listed these in Table 2 and briefly discuss each below.

Patient-Individual Practitioner Interaction

The care provided by a practitioner to a patient is the fundamental interaction in health care. Here, the individual characteristics of a patient are addressed by a practitioner with a unique mix of knowledge, experience, technical skill, and interpersonal skill.

15

Of the four units of analysis, the patient-practitioner interaction has received the most attention in the quality assurance literature. Whether measured in terms of the accuracy of the diagnosis or the appropriateness and effectiveness of treatment, the subject of most quality assurance studies has been the care provided by a practitioner to a patient. Likewise, much of the literature on patient satisfaction addresses the patient's assessment of, accessibility to, and sense of comfort with his or her clinician.

What are the determinants of the quality of this patient-practitioner? A partial listing might include:

1). Accurate and complete description by the patient of health problems and care needs;

2). Accurate history-taking and physical examination and proper synthesis of this information by the practitioner;

3). Appropriate ordering of diagnostic tests and accurate analysis and use of their results;

4). Appropriate use of efficacious therapeutic modalities and appropriate monitoring of their effectiveness;

5). Appropriate education by the practitioner of the patient and family concerning the nature of the health problem, the planned treatment, and necessary preventive measures; and

6). Compliance by the patient with the treatment regimen and timely and accurate reporting of the patient's perception of the treatment's degree of effectiveness.

These parameters of quality are important both individually and collectively and emphasize the fact that optimal clinical outcomes are dependent upon the joint, ongoing effort of patients and their clinicians.

Patient-Practitioner Team Interaction

Often overlooked in the quality assurance literature, the nature of the interaction between an individual patient and multiple practitioners is now being recognized as a central determinant of quality. Knaus and his colleagues, in an important examination of the quality of care in intensive care units (ICU), demonstrated that differences in quality among ICUs appeared to relate primarily to the degree to which the ICU team worked together effectively.[15] This finding is discussed further in Chapter 4.

The importance of effective interaction between practitioners is not restricted to the high technology, labor intensive environment of an ICU. Treatment of the severely chronically mentally ill, when done well, involves the physician, the psychologist, the nurse, the social worker, and often occupational, physical, and speech therapists to help the individual achieve incremental improvement in social, physical, and occupational skills. The composition of such teams varies over time and by patient. It is, however, a rare patient with severe chronic mental illness who does not need the services of such a team at various times in the course of the illness. Likewise, one can highlight the importance to quality of the coordinated work, for example, of the surgeon and internist in the case of a patient with severe diabetes requiring major surgery, or the physician, home care nurse, and cleric in coordinated attention to the physical, psychological, and spiritual needs of a terminally ill patient.

Complementing the determinants of quality for the one-to-one patient-individual practitioner interaction, one can enumerate the characteristics of quality in the interaction among a team of practitioners. These characteristics include:

1). Timely and accurate communication of patient-specific information and changes in diagnostic or therapeutic approaches;

2). Effective synthesis of information coming from multiple sources, each having a somewhat different view of the patient and a different capability and responsibility to evaluate and treat the patient; and

3). Effective coordination of both the personal interaction with the patient and the diagnostic and therapeutic interventions used to help the patient.

The Health Care Organization

The next unit of analysis for evaluating quality is the health care organization. Of the four "units of analysis," the health care organization rivals the patient-practitioner interaction in the degree of attention it has received. This attention has resulted from the fact that purchasers of health care in the past have often looked, and in the future will increasingly look, to organizations, not individual practitioners, for contracts for the provision of care. This tendency is well illustrated by the emphasis that the Health Care Financing Administration, U.S. Department of Health and Human Services, has placed on the expansion of HMO/CMP risk contracting in Medicare. (See Chapters 5 and 9.) It also can be seen in the emphasis business and private insurers have given to offering managed care plans to their employees or enrollees. Purchasers and those they represent, having stimulated expansion in health care plans, now face an often bewildering array of plans from which to chose. To inform their selection, they are now seeking information on the quality of each plan.

Earlier in this chapter, I listed a set of organizational characteristics believed to help assure quality. To illustrate the importance of these characteristics, consider the relevance of one of them, clarity of organizational purpose, implicit in the remarkably different missions of the following hospitals: a metropolitan, public, general hospital; a university hospital; a medium-size, community hospital in an affluent suburb; and a rural hospital serving a small, isolated town. The public hospital must often organize itself to assure adequate care to a largely uninsured population. Many university hospitals must remember that they are not only tertiary referral institutions, but also hospitals providing routine care. Thus, they must assure the capability to meet both the most complex and the most mundane of health care needs. The community hospital must understand the limits of its ability to support the technological desires of a large number of practitioners and devote its attention to those services which the community truly needs and which it can provide in a competent fashion. The rural hospital must balance the pressures that its remote setting creates to expand service capability with a realistic understanding of the limitations in the economic resources and clinical competences available to do so.

Beyond this very basic requirement for clarity of organizational purpose is the need for the organization, a hospital in this case, to create a physical, human-resource, and management environment which is safe for patients and employees and which fosters effective patient care. Specific characteristics needed to achieve such safe and effective care include competence in governance and management, coordination of services across time, care settings, and organizations, and proven, reliable quality control and assurance mechanisms.

The trend toward increasing regional and national consolidation of health care organizations further complicates the evaluation of quality at the organizational level. Fully one-third of all hospital beds are now in hospitals which are members of multi-unit systems with another major component involved in consortiums of various types. The influence these organizations have over the quality of care within individual hospitals differs from one system to another. Their influence is not negligible, however, and should be considered when one is evaluating the quality of care provided by a system hospital.

The Community

Health care in this country has been distinctly local in its flavor. Whether one is considering differences in the organization of care or the variation between localities in practice patterns, we see tremendous differences in the local health care arrangements across this country. The growth of regional and national health systems, the development of national contracts to provide comprehensive care, and the movement away from the courts' acceptance of local standards of care will undoubtedly temper, but not eliminate, the importance of attending to the particular health care needs of each community.

The forces pushing for competition and efficiency in health care have not been without impact, however, on the delivery of local health care. Whereas local health care was once dominated by the physician and hospital, we now see the growing influence of the purchasers and insurers of care, and the appearance of health plans which encompass both the insurance and delivery aspects of health care. Where once it was clear that the physician and hospital were responsible for quality, we now see a diffusion and extension of this responsibility. This diffusion has prompted many communities to create coalitions to impose some order on the rapid change entailed in this largely unanticipated, albeit incremental, restructuring of their local health care. From such concern has come a reawakening of interest in both better defining community health care needs and measuring how well these needs are being met. This interest, if implemented appropriately, will create pressure to restructure community health care to better address identified problems.

Out of this evolving scenario, what can be identified as the central ingredients of quality at the community level? The following would appear important:

1). Identifying the health care and preventive care needs of the community;

2). Assuring the availability of, and accessibility to, needed care; and

3). Assuring continuity of care across practitioner and organization.

IDENTIFYING INDICATORS OF QUALITY

To this point, I have described the seven key elements of quality health care and four possible units of analysis which could be examined in a quality evaluation program. Combining these two approaches creates the four-by-six matrix shown in Table 3.

Within the cells of this matrix can be placed indicators used to monitor the quality of care. What might be the characteristics of these indicators? What aspects of care might they measure? In answering these questions, it is well to start with Donabedian's classic triad of structure, process, and outcome.[16] In Donabedian's construct, structural measures address the characteristics of the setting in which care is provided and of the individual(s) providing or supporting care. Thus, such measures would assess the nature of the organizational and physical environment, the types of technology available for diagnosis and treatment, and the number, type, and qualifications of the professionals providing the care. Process measures specify the elements of the care delivered. They encompass preventive, diagnostic, therapeutic, and maintenance clinical activities, as well as the managerial procedures attendant to that care. Outcome measures assess the consequences of health care. They can include projected levels of physical or psychological functioning; survival rates; and the nature and incidence of complications of care.

Thus, for each cell (for instance, individual professional competence in the patient-practitioner interaction), one could identify indicators related to structure, process, or outcome. For example, if one is interested in the competence of physicians in the management of diabetes, one could utilize: 1) *structural indicators* such as board certification and duration of training in the care of diabetics; 2) *process indicators* such as effective use of laboratory tests; or

20

3) *outcome indicators* such as incidence of severe hyperglycemia or hypoglycemia, incidence of hospitalization for a practitioner's diabetic patients, or the rapidity of control of blood glucose.

Taking the structure, process, and outcome concept one step further, it is often appropriate to subcategorize indicators into clinical and administrative groups. Such classification is particularly important when one is attempting to differentiate the degree to which either the practitioner or the organizational support system contributes to or hinders delivery of quality care.

This distinction between practitioner and organization can be illustrated by considering the care of the diabetic patient in a severe hyperglycemic coma. To analyze the quality of care provided in this situation, one may choose to utilize indicators related to the competence both of the specific practitioners treating the patient and of those who have designed and now operate the administrative systems supporting the clinician. In this analysis, one could use, for the former, one or more of the clinically oriented indicators noted before (board certification, adequacy of lab testing, and rapidity of control of block glucose levels) and, for the latter, administrative indicators such as the ability to access existence of "stat" serum glucose testing (structure), timely turnaround of serum glucose test results (process), and consistently accurate testing results (outcome).

While it is desirable to identify indicators related to specific aspects of the quality of care received by a patient or a group of patients, it is often not possible to do so. For instance, an outcome measure such as the rapidity of control of a patient with severly abnormal blood glucose tests the competence of the practitioner, the health care team, and those managing the hospital. The more general the indicator, the less powerful will be its attribution capability.

A further example of this problem can be found in the recent release to the public of hospital-specific mortality rates for Medicare beneficiaries.[17] Are these data useful as measures of the quality of care provided by hospitals in this country? In my view, in their current state, they are not. First, death is most often not due to poor care, but is the natural result of the end stages of a disease process. Beyond this, however, is the fact that the Medicare data are flawed in several ways. First, there is inadequate accounting for the differences which exist in the severity of the illness among the patient populations cared for in the different hospitals. Severity adjustment is discussed in Chapters 2 and 3, so I will not discuss it further here. Suffice it to say here that the lack of such adjustment renders these data invalid as a measure of quality.

Further, the data suffer from the problem of lumping. In the Medicare release, data were aggregated into 16 groups, each encompassing a large number of DRG categories. Yet mortality rates (and most often other outcome indicators) increase in their power to unearth quality problems the more narrowly their content is defined. Thus, one learns more from knowing cancer death rates than from knowing total hospital mortality rates; more from Hodgkins disease death rates than from overall cancer death rates; and more from Hodgkins disease death rates by stage than from overall Hodgkins death rates. Thus, we would be better served by the release of data for more specific diagnostic categories appropriately adjusted for severity.

To return now to the categorization of indicators, Table 3 presents a quality evaluation matrix which identifies the major cells into which indicators can be placed. Table 4 illustrates that for any one of the cells in Table 3, one can categorize indicators by their structure, process, or outcome orientation. (Professional competence is used as the example in this table.) Finally, Table 5 demonstrates that structure, process, and outcome indicators can be of either a clinical or an administrative nature.

THE BASIC ELEMENTS OF
A QUALITY EVALUATION PROGRAM

Having proceeded from a definition of quality care to the description of a classification system for indicators of quality, I will now outline the optimal characteristics of programs which utilize these indicators to evaluate quality.

For this discussion, I draw from the Joint Commission's experience in developing standards for quality assurance programs. The evolution of our thinking on quality assurance is described in more detail elsewhere and has been synthesized into a "generic model" for monitoring and evaluating the quality of care.[18] This model is outlined in Table 6 and includes ten steps necessary to assure that the program will be priority-focused, efficient, and effective. In this discussion, I will focus on hospitals, but the content of the discussion can be generalized to almost any type of health care organization.

We start with the notion that the responsibility for the program must be clearly assigned. Responsibility for quality evaluation resides at several levels of a hospital (governance, senior management, departmental leadership, medical and support staff). The division of responsibility among these parties will vary somewhat from hospital to hospital and should be clearly stated in the hospital's formal documents (bylaws, policies, procedures). With such responsibility must come the commitment to quality which is essential for excellence in patient care.

The next step is to gain a clear understanding of the specific nature of the clinical care provided by the hospital or department: what conditions, diagnoses, or clinical problems are treated, and what diagnostic or therapeutic services are rendered? Clear articulation of the scope of services can then be used to begin the priority-setting processes which will serve to focus attention on those areas of care which are most important to monitor.

Step Three involves the selection from the full scope of services those which are most critical to monitor. Particular attention should be given to services that are high-volume, high-risk, or that otherwise may be prone to quality problems. Examples of problem-prone services include those that are new, are felt intuitively to be a problem, or that have some tangible but as yet inconclusive data indicating the presence of a problem.

The next step is to identify for each of these aspects of care indicators or measures of quality that encompass as many of the seven characteristics of quality noted in Table 1 as possible and are related to clinical or administrative structure, process, or outcomes (Tables 3, 4, and 5). For each of these indicators, it is best to identify the levels of acceptable and unacceptable performance (step 5) and focus further attention on those areas found to be outside of the acceptable level. For example, a hospital may have chosen to monitor post-operative nosocomial infection rates--a clinical outcome indicator. It is well recognized that such infections will occur in even the best of hospitals. Thus, while each infection must be handled clinically, it is important not to waste precious quality assurance resources on investigation of the quality of care in each case. Rather, one should investigate the quality of infection control procedures in detail only if the rate exceeds a predetermined standard (e.g., 3 percent of operative procedures). By contrast, there are outcomes that are unusual enough such that each occurrence should be analyzed. Such "sentinel events" are illustrated by an outcome such as a maternal death during or immediately following delivery. In this case, the threshold is not a rate but the occurrence itself. (See Chapter 2 for a further discussion of "sentinel events.")

The next two steps relate to the collection and analysis of data. Effective quality assurance depends upon the identification and definition of the necessary data elements and the appropriate assignment of responsibility for the data gathering and management.

The evaluation of data usually involves a screening process in which a comparison is made with preestablished standards followed by further evaluation of any care falling outside the threshold. Where warranted, the care is then subject to review by peers examining the full clinical context of the case or cases in question. The importance of objective, clinically relevant peer review cannot be overemphasized. The technology of quality assurance has not progressed to the point where any single indicator is powerful enough to discriminate good care from bad. This distinction can only be accomplished by the objective evaluation of peers. (See Chapter 2.)

Step Eight is an obvious but often neglected responsibility. To improve quality, one must constantly enhance performance in areas of clinical or organizational weakness. If such improvement is not possible, the individual or organization must cease providing the care in question. To date, the need to correct problems has often been slowed by fear of liability, reluctance to confront a peer, and concern over the economic consequences of adverse decisions to the hospital or referring colleagues. Such problems are receiving positive attention through the courts and, in certain instances, through legislation itself.[19] (See Chapter 13.)

Step Nine entails the need to evaluate the results of corrective actions. This step is important in so far as it is often not possible to pin-point the precise cause of a problem. In such instances, one should undertake the corrective measures and then monitor the indicator data closely. These data will often provide the information needed to assure whether the action taken was effective.

Finally, it is important to recognize that quality assurance activities should not, and cannot effectively, operate in a vacuum. Their findings can and should be used in decisions involving privilege delineation, in analysis of a hospital's or a department's range of services, and to assess other departments which may be contributing unknowingly to poor quality care.

PUTTING IT ALL TOGETHER

In the preceding sections of this chapter, I have attempted to describe the components needed to construct an effective quality evaluation effort. The essential ingredients are: 1) a clear view of the fundamental goal or purpose of health care; 2) a definition of the major characteristics of care which are necessary to achieve this purpose; 3) identification of the component(s) of the health care system one wishes to analyze; 4) a knowledgeable selection of the indicators to be utilized; and 5) a process by which the evaluation occurs.

To illustrate the relevance and flexibility of this model, consider again the evaluation of the quality of care of those with cancer. In my statement of the purpose of health care, I have indicated that one should identify and effectively address the educational, preventive, restorative, and maintenance needs of patients. In a quality evaluation program, one could choose to examine any one or all of these possible needs.

For the care addressed to any one of these needs, it would be possible to analyze the availability/accessibility, appropriateness, acceptability, continuity, professional competence, or safety of that care. Further, any of these characteristics of care could be examined using the patient-practitioner, patient-team, organization, or community as the unit of analysis. Similarly, for any of these four units of analysis, one could identify and evaluate clinical and administrative indicators of structure, process, and outcome.

Finally, the process of evaluation is most effective if integrated into a system of quality assurance which is structured, accountable, objective, and effective. The flow of this overall system of quality assurance is illustrated in Figure 1 and is applicable to programs operating in a hospital, group practice, nursing home, mental health clinic, hospice program, home care agency, managed care plan, or any other health care organization.

Table 1

Elements of High Quality Care

1. Availability
2. Accessibility
3. Appropriateness
4. Acceptability
5. Continuity
6. Professional competence
7. Physical safety

Table 2

Four Possible Units of Analysis in Evaluating Quality

1. Patient-individual practitioner interaction
2. Patient-practitioner team interaction
3. Health care organization
4. Health care community

Table 3

The Quality Evaluation Matrix

Elements of Quality

	Availability/ accessibility	Appropriateness	Acceptability	Continuity	Professional competence	Physical safety
Patient-individual practitioner interaction						
Patient-practitioner team interaction						
Health care organization						
Health care community						

vertical -- Units of Analysis

Table 4

Types of Quality Indicators by Element of Quality:
The Example of Professional Competence

Element of Quality: Professional Competence

Structure	
Type of Indicator — Process	
Outcome	

Table 5

Further Differentiating Indicators

Subject of the Indicator

	Clinical	Administrative
Structure		
Process		
Outcome		

Type of Indicator

Table 6

The Ten Step "Generic" Model
for Monitoring and Evaluating the Quality of Care

Step	Activity
#1	Assign responsibility for each component of the program.
#2	Delineate the types of clinical care provided.
#3	Identify the most important aspects of care.
#4	Identify indicator related to those aspects of care.
#5	Establish thresholds for evaluation for each indicator.
#6	Collect and organize data related to the indicators.
#7	Evaluate care when thresholds are reached.
#8	Take actions to improve care.
#9	Assess the effectiveness of the actions.
#10	Communicate relevant information to others in the organization.

**Figure 1. An overall system of quality assurance:
the steps in the development of the system.**

Clear statement of the
purpose or goal of care

Identification of major
characteristics of high
quality care

Identification of the
units of analysis

Specification of quality
indicators

Integration of these measures
into quality evaluation program

NOTES

1. R.M. Pirsig, *Zen and the Art of Motorcycle Maintenance* (New York: Bantam Books, 1974).

2. E.W. Deming, *Out of the Crisis* (Cambridge, MA: Massachusetts Institute of Technology, 1986).

3. P.B. Crosby, *Quality is Free* (New York: Menton Books, New American Library, 1979).

4. J.E. Wennberg, "The Medical Care Outcome Problem: An Agenda for Action," paper presented at National Leadership Commission on Health Care, Washington, DC, 1987.

5. D.M. Eddy, and J. Billings, "The Quality of Medical Evidence and Medical Practice," paper presented at National Leadership Commission on Health Care, Washington, DC, 1987.

6. E. Vayda, "A Comparison of Surgical Rates in Canada and in England and Wales," *New England Journal of Medicine* 289(1973): 1224-1229.

7. J.E. Wennberg, N.P. Roos, L. Sola, et al., "Use of Claims Data Systems to Evaluate Health Care Outcomes: Mortality and Reoperation Following Prostatectomy," *Journal of the American Medical Association*, 257(1987): 933-936.

8. C.E. Lewis, "Variations in the Incidence of Surgery," *New England Journal of Medicine*, 281(1969): 880-884.

9. J.D. Wennberg and A. Gittellsohn, "Small Area Variations in Health Care Delivery," *Science*, 182(1973): 1102-1108.

10. *Confronting Regional Variation: The Maine Approach* (Chicago, IL: American Medical Association, 1986).

11. R.W. DuBois, R.H. Brook, and Wh.H. Rogers, "Adjusted Hospital Death Rates: A Potential Screen for Quality of Medical Care," *American Journal of Public Health*, 77(1987): 1162-1166.

12. N.J. Merrick, R.H. Brook, A. Fink, and D.H. Solomon, "Use of Carotid Endarterectomy in Five California Veterans Administration Medical Centers," *Journal of the American Medical Association*, 256(1986): 2531.

13. S. Shortell, Northwestern University, personal communication.

14. E.R. Camplin, O.R. Keil, A. McLean, J. Ness, and K.M. Tomasik, *Hazardous Waste Management: Controlling Asbestos and Waste Anesthesia Gases* (Chicago, IL:, Joint Commission on Accreditation of Healthcare Organizations, 1987).

15. W.A. Knaus, E.A. Dragon, D.P. Wagner, and J.E. Zimmerman, "An Evaluation of Outcome From Intensive Care in Major Medical Centers, *Annals of Internal Medicine*, 104(1986): 410.

16. A. Donabedian, *A Guide to Medical Administration, Vol. II, Medical Care Appraisal--Quality and Utilization* (Washington, DC: American Public Health Association, 1969).

17. *Medicare Hospital Mortality Information, 1986* (Washington, DC: Health Care Financing Administration, Department of Health and Human Services, December, 1987).

18. J.S. Roberts and R.M. Walczak, "Quality Assurance: The Evolution and Current Status of the Joint Commission on Accreditation of Hospitals, Quality Assurance Standard," *Quality Review Bulletin* 10(1984): 11-15.

19. Title IV PL 99-660, "Healthcare Quality Improvement Act of 1986."

Chapter 2

Quantifying Quality

Christy Moynihan, Ph.D.

The recent emphasis on quality in the delivery of health care has focused attention on techniques for measuring quality. There has been substantial progress in our ability to measure quality in recent years, and this progress will undoubtedly continue given the amount of research currently underway in this area. This chapter gives an overview of the methods currently in use or under development to measure quality. It attempts to explain the appropriate use of each method, its strengths and weaknesses, and its potential for further development.

Approaches for measuring quality are commonly classified as addressing one of three dimensions: structure, process, or outcome. (See Chapter 1.) This chapter will focus only on process and out-come-oriented methods. In describing these methods, however, we will use a somewhat different classification system based on the meth-odological approach used in the assessment. As shown in Figure 1, we distinguish two fundamental methodological approaches to quality assessment: one based on individual case review and another based on statistical analysis. Although the distinction can be blurred, the former is essentially process-based, while the latter is outcome-ori-ented. As will be shown, these two methodological approaches are complementary. In the long run, it is probably necessary to use a blend of both to achieve truly meaningful results.

THE TWO METHODOLOGICAL APPROACHES
TO QUALITY ASSESSMENT

The first of the two methodological approaches, case review, is defined as the evaluation of care provided to individual patients. This evaluation may entail direct observation or medical record review. In case review, care is evaluated in relationship to clinical norms which reflect recognized standards of care. These norms may be subjective ("implicit criteria"). Ideally, however, they are formulated as "explicit criteria" developed specifically for the clinical area under review. Using the case review methodology, it is possible to assign a judgment to the care rendered to a single patient. Thus, it is possible to state, for example, that patient X received appropriate care or substandard care at hospital Y during his admission for diagnosis Z.

Statistical assessment, on the other hand, does not depend upon the use of clinical norms. It allows for the measurement of quality through comparison with statistical norms or "expected values." For example, by using statistical analysis for examining mortality rates across hospitals, one can identify hospitals for which the mortality rate is higher or lower than expected, given the hospital's patient mix. Statistical assessment cannot assign a judgment to the care rendered to an individual patient, however. It can only infer that, over a group of cases, patients in hospital Y, on average, received acceptable care or poor quality care either in the aggregate or for certain types of clinical services. Statistical methods are thus always comparative (e.g., comparing hospital Y with a national or regional norm). Results from case review that provide information on individual patients may also be aggregated to yield comparative data.

Other differences between the case review approach and the statistical approach include the following. The case review approach is generally manual and often entails the collection of primary data. The statistical approach is computerized. As a result, the case review approach has a relatively high cost per case and thus is often confined to use with a "small" number of cases. The statistical approach, however, lends itself well to examination of a large number of cases and thus is often able to detect subtle differences in care among hospitals, physicians, or regions that might not be apparent from a small number of cases.

When evaluating any quality measurement or classification system, researchers are concerned with both validity (the extent to which the measurement accurately reflects the properties of the item being measured) and reliability (the reproducibility of the measurements made, i.e., the degree to which measurements taken at two different times or by two different people agree). Case review criteria often have a high degree of clinical specificity. That is, the conclusion reached in evaluating a specific case is generally made on the basis of careful consideration of the unique clinical details of the case. The conclusion should, therefore, validly reflect the care given to the patient. Because of the ultimate reliance in the case review method on subjective clinical judgment, however, two people reviewing the same case with the same criteria may arrive at two different conclusions. Thus, reliability can suffer.

Statistical analysis, on the other hand, poses difficulty in terms of acceptable validity because of its reliance on existing data sources. Two people using the same data and computer programs may arrive at the same conclusion and therefore achieve high reliability, but the conclusion could well be wrong. For example, there may be so many errors in the coding of the patients' admitting diagnoses that they obviate valid conclusions from the statistical analysis. Even straightforward outcomes of the treatment episode, such as mortality, may not be reliably coded in the data.

Within the two basic approaches to measuring quality, case review and statistical analysis, there are different specific methods. These methods are listed in Figure 2. As shown, the case review approach encompasses two methods, termed "diagnosis-specific" and "generic." Statistical analysis also encompasses two approaches, termed "controlled" and "nonexperimental."

UTILIZATION REVIEW VERSUS QUALITY ASSESSMENT

Before beginning our discussion of these methods, it would appear worthwhile to distinguish between the measurement of quality and utilization review (UR). The two concepts are closely related, but they are not identical. A confusion of utilization review methods with quality assessment tools will only serve to complicate an already complex issue. Utilization review is the evaluation of care in terms of the appropriateness of the level of services provided. The aspects of utilization most commonly focused on are the necessity of an acute hospital admission and the necessity of invasive procedures. Appropriate utilization is a component of quality care, but quality is not limited to utilization. For instance, underutilization is certainly a quality problem. Failing to hospitalize a patient who requires acute services or discharging one prematurely is poor quality care. Similarly, overutilization is also a quality problem, since providing any service, even bed rest in a hospital, presents some iatrogenic risk to the patient. Providing unnecessary services presents unnecessary risk, with the degree of risk increasing with the invasiveness of the service provided. Established UR criteria are therefore useful in assessing the aspects of quality that relate to both under- and over-utilization. The concept of quality, however, is broader and encompasses attributes of all treatment decisions regarding the patient, not just those relating to level of care and provision of invasive procedures. (See Chapter 1.)

Utilization-based analyses are sometimes proposed as a means of quality assessment. Such studies can be misleading, however. Utilization measures used as care standards are essentially process measures. They are valid as a quality indicator only when a clinical consensus has been established concerning the appropriate frequency or intensity level of the service or procedure in question. Small area analysis of hospital utilization rates is a case in point. (See Chapter 8.) By examining utilization rates in contiguous areas, this method is able to detect areas in which rates are deviant, either much higher or much lower than average. Such studies are currently being promoted as quality assessment methodologies.

While these methods can effectively identify variations in practice, they cannot by themselves identify which is the appropriate standard of practice. Under certain extreme circumstances, it may be obvious that utilization rates in an area are too low and reflect inadequate access and low quality of care or are too high and reflect overutilization. In general, however, the volume of hospital services needed to promote optimum health outcomes has not yet been established.[1] The examination of practice variations, in fact, calls out for a more direct assessment of their relationship to quality of care, using the methods to be discussed below. (See, for example, two recent studies concerning appropriate rates for carotid endarterectomy.[2,3])

CASE REVIEW METHODS OF QUALITY ASSESSMENT

Diagnosis-Specific Approaches

Characteristics of diagnosis-specific approaches

The diagnosis-specific approach could well be the oldest approach to assessing quality and was at the heart of the Medical Care Evaluation studies used by Professional Standards Review Organizations

(PSROs) to measure quality. This approach is based on the premise that the care provided depends upon the patient's problem or condition and that determining the quality of care provided a patient cannot be accomplished without first defining appropriate standards of care for the patient's condition.

To implement the diagnosis-specific approach, the investigator first identifies a set of conditions on which to focus the review. These may be areas in which there are known or suspected quality-of-care problems. Once the conditions are selected, normative standards for treatment of the condition are developed through examination of the literature and/or through the use of a panel of experts. These standards are then expressed in clear written form for use by physician or nonphysician reviewers.

The criteria are most often expressed in "list" form (see Figure 3). The list specifies a set of procedures which should always be performed for a patient with a given diagnosis. Greenfield et al. have shown, however, that criteria may have greater predictive power when they are in "map" form; i.e., they follow the clinical decision-making process by specifying which actions should be performed contingent upon the results of prior actions.[4] This latter approach has not been widely adopted, however.

Strengths and weaknesses

The diagnosis-specific approach can achieve high levels of validity when the standards are developed and applied properly. The approach can also yield a continuous score for the quality of care provided, ranging from superior to grossly substandard. This attribute allows for the identification of marginally suboptimal care as well as that which is frankly substandard. Some of the other approaches to be discussed below tend to focus on a fairly narrow range of frankly substandard care and lack the sensitivity to detect the marginally suboptimal.

The disadvantage of the diagnosis-specific approach is that it is costly, both to develop the criteria and to apply them. Thus, the diagnosis-specific approach tends to focus on a relatively small number of diagnostic categories. Kessner et al., however, attempted to illustrate how a limited set of diagnoses or "tracer conditions" could serve as an adequate proxy for a much broader range of care given by a provider.[5] If an investigator's goal is to use tracer conditions to provide a broad assessment of the quality of a given institution, facility, or even a health care system, the tracers must be carefully chosen to provide the maximum coverage and impact. To make a general assessment of a facility, the investigator may prefer to select as tracers a sample of conditions which are relatively common, for which there are well-established standards, and for which failure to adhere to standards has fairly severe consequences.

A final feature of the diagnosis-specific approach which can be both an advantage and a disadvantage is that it focuses primarily on process. This focus has the advantage of allowing the investigator to make more detailed judgments about quality than possible with other methods to be described primarily because it allows an in-depth examination of the treatment decisions made throughout an episode of care. However, as with process measures in general, it is often difficult to quantify the clinical impact of deviations from the established standards. Almost all cases fail to meet at least one of the standards. It is difficult, however, to tell in an absolute sense how serious the failure is in terms of actual or potential harm to the patient.

As a result of these considerations, the primary uses of the diagnosis-specific approach are for focused review (i.e., review which is targeted on known or potential problem areas) and research. The method may be particularly suited to ongoing use in a clinical setting over time, for example, for use by a hospital's quality assurance department or by a medical school in evaluating the effectiveness of its clinical training programs. The clinical specificity of the information gleaned in the review makes the method particularly applicable to the monitoring and correcting of individual practitioner performance. It is not, however, a realistic approach for widescale monitoring.

Generic Case Review

Characteristics of generic case review

Generic approaches to quality assessment are partially a response to the need for tools which apply more widely than diagnosis-specific approaches, and, unlike the latter, can be used to evaluate all, rather than a sample, of generic case review cases for a given health care institution or system. Generic approaches to quality assessment, as their name implies, replace the diagnosis-specific criteria with a single "generic" set of criteria which can be applied uniformly across all diagnostic categories. They do this by shifting the emphasis in the review. Whereas diagnosis-specific approaches identify what should occur in providing care for a given diagnostic entity, generic approaches define what should *not* occur in treating any patient. Generic approaches are thus oriented to the identification of adverse occurrences; i.e., poor health outcomes which, when they occur, have a high probability of association with substandard care.

This approach, also termed "adverse occurrence screening," owes much of its development to the work of Joyce Craddick, M.D.[6] Craddick's chart review system flags cases that evidence certain untoward patient events or adverse patient occurrences which are not a natural consequence of the patient's disease. These include such events as:

- admission for complications or adverse results of out-patient management;

- unplanned removal, injury, or repair of organ or structure during surgery, invasive procedure, or vaginal delivery;

- neurological deficit present at discharge which was not present on admission; and

- unexpected death.

Charts that fail to pass the screens are then subjected to more intensive review by a physician reviewer to determine whether or not the adverse event was avoidable and due to a deficiency in the care provided. The approach was recently mandated by the Health Care Financing Administration (HCFA) for use by the nation's 54 peer review organizations in their second contract period. (See Chapters 5,6, and 9.) The six HCFA generic screens, presented in Figure 4, are similar to those developed by Craddick. Like Craddick's screens, the HCFA screens are oriented to actual observable adverse events.

The generic screen criteria currently in use are for assessing inpatient care. A similar concept underlies the method now being used by PROs in their review of the quality of care in HMOs. In this method, admission to the hospital in an advanced stage of disease is viewed as an adverse outcome that may indicate a deficiency in the quality of prior outpatient care. (See Chapter 9.) In Chapter 3, Gonnella and Louis similarly discuss the occurrence of "late-stage" admissions as a possible signal of poor outpatient care.

Such types of generic measures recall the work of Rutstein et al. who developed the concept of "sentinel events"; i.e., "cases of unnecessary disease and unnecessary disability, and unnecessary untimely deaths [whose] occurrence is a warning signal, a sentinel event, that the quality of care may need to be improved."[7] Rutstein et al. proposed as sentinel events such measures as deaths from cervical cancer, low birth weight, and other outcomes preventable through effective health system monitoring. While they intended these measures to be used as part of a nationwide statistical monitoring system rather than as a case review method, sentinel events can be used like Craddick's adverse occurrences to select cases in an HMO or other self-contained health system for further review to determine whether these events reflect deficiencies in the care provided.

Strengths and weaknesses

Generic screening allows for efficient review across the whole spectrum of diseases, not just selected diagnoses. It also increases the efficiency of the review process by concentrating on the most serious quality defects; i.e., those that have resulted in actual harm to the patient. The approach allows for widescale monitoring by, for example, PROs. It is useful for the same reason in hospital quality-assurance and risk-management departments. Like the diagnosis-specific approach, it is based on review of the medical record or other case documentation. It, therefore, produces the clinical detail needed to change individual behavior.

As stated above, the major strength of generic screening systems in their pure form is their concentration on actual adverse occurrences. This strength is also a major weakness. Serious deficiencies in the care rendered to a patient can have the "potential" for causing significant harm but not result in actual harm to the patient. For example, a physician's failure to biopsy a breast mass in a specific patient may not result in actual harm to that patient because a 75 percent probability exists that the mass is benign.[8] A consistent failure by a physician to perform any biopsies when discovering new breast masses, however, is a serious care deficiency because the delay in diagnosis and treatment will compromise the outcome for the 25 percent of the patients in whom the breast mass is malignant.

A truly comprehensive approach would uncover these deficiencies as well as those resulting in actual harm. The developers of generic systems seem to recognize the need to detect deficiencies which produce no actual harm, but have the potential for harm. For instance, one of the HCFA generic screens reads as follows:

Adverse drug reaction or medication error with *serious potential for harm* [emphasis added], or resulting in special measures to correct (e.g., intubation, cardio-pulmonary resuscitation, gastric lavage)...

Unlike observable adverse occurrences, the detection of medication errors with "serious potential for harm" requires a greater knowledge of appropriate indications, contraindications and therapeutic ranges for drugs. Such errors may not be easily detected in a routine screening of the patient's record. In general, effective identification of problems with potential rather than actual harm requires a strong process orientation which in turn requires criteria with greater specificity than found in generic screening sets. The HCFA generic screens and other generic screening systems, therefore, rely heavily on the clinical judgment of the reviewers, a fact which may make them more unreliable in identifying process errors than a diagnosis-specific approach.

An additional problem with the generic screening approach is that the identification of an adverse occurrence; e.g., death during or closely following elective surgery, does not necessarily signify that a quality problem actually occurred. To determine whether or not one did, the chart must be examined by a physician using clinical judgment in areas that are often very specialized and may be highly subjective as well. Unlike the well delineated standards in the diagnosis-specific approaches, however, process standards may not be developed for this specific chart review and may have to be left to the clinical judgment of the physician reviewer--a fact, which introduces subjectivity into, and reduces both the validity and reliability of, the review process.

Even with chart review, it may be difficult to ascertain whether a given adverse outcome is truly the result of a deficiency in the care provided. Nosocomial infections and death during high-risk operations occur in every hospital. Therefore, their presence in a given institution does not per se constitute poor quality. It is when there is a disproportionate number of these occurrences for a given facility or physician that one infers poor quality of care. Thus, examination of individual cases must at some point be wedded to statistical systems to evaluate and monitor quality of care effectively.

Generic screening, which has been discussed above as a manual case review system, can, in fact, be implemented as an automated system. At this point, it begins to blend with statistical approaches. Like statistical approaches, generic screening is outcome oriented. In implementing a manual screening system, the reviewer examines the medical record for adverse outcomes. If a hospital data system is comprehensive enough and incorporates a sufficient number of specific codes to describe all signficant clinical events that may occur during a stay, the screens can be integrated into the data system to flag automatically cases which have indicators of the adverse events. If such a system is used only to flag individual cases which are then subjected to further review, it is functioning merely as an automated version of the manual process. However, if the system is also used to aggregate cases to identify deviant patterns by service or physician, for example, then it is also functioning as a statistical system.

This concept is the basis of the system currently under development by the Joint Commission on Accreditation of Healthcare Organizations (JCAHO) to introduce clinical indicators into the process of accrediting hospitals. (See Chapter 1.) The JCAHO proposes to use indicators such as nosocomial infection rates, internal transfers to an intensive care unit, surgical complication rates, discrepancies in pathology reports, fourth-degree tears for obstetrical patients, and so forth. Rather than using these to focus review on individual cases, however, the system will be a purely statistical one, as described in the following statement:

> Data relative to specified indicators would be routinely and continuously collected by departments throughout the institution, an activity which should be occurring now under current quality assurance standards. At regular

intervals throughout the period of accreditation, clinical and organizational data would be submitted to the Joint Commission either in writing, or by PC diskette, or by data tape, or perhaps even by modem... [9]

The JCAHO would process the data and provide feedback to the institution so it could compare its performance to its expectations, as an "early warning system," and to external expectations based on national performance standards.

To sum, generic screening is a case review method which focuses review by identifying cases with actual adverse outcomes. Once a case is identified, further record review is required to determine whether there has been a deficiency in the process of care. Generic screening is useful, therefore, for covering a wide range of clinical situations, including those which may be too complex to permit development of more specific process measures. It also focuses review on cases with the worst outcomes. Unlike diagnosis-specific approaches, identification of process errors with potential, but no actual, harm is not accommodated within this approach. Both the diagnosis-specific and generic screening approaches have one common characteristic. Neither can be appropriately used unless: 1) the correct diagnostic and therapeutic process for the case under review has been established, and 2) it is possible through review of the documentation for the case to determine whether that process was adhered to. When these conditions are not met, statistical approaches become the most feasible method of evaluating quality.

STATISTICAL APPROACHES TO ASSESSING QUALITY

Statistical approaches infer that the process of care is appropriate or deficient by detecting outcomes that are statistically equivalent to or worse than expected over a large number of cases. Statistical approaches thus do not require an intensive review of the process of care as case review methods do. Statistical methods are, in fact, often used to determine whether certain processes or aspects of the care rendered have a beneficial or deleterious effect on outcome. The major problem with statistical approaches is that there are many other factors beside the one under consideration that may affect the outcome. It is often difficult to be certain that all of these other factors have been accounted for.

The statistical approach to quality assessment is currently an area of substantial interest primarily due to the implementation of the Prospective Payment System (PPS) in Medicare. Statistical analysis is less expensive than the case review methods and is the only feasible method for performing the wide scale monitoring and evaluation needed to assess the possibly subtle impacts of PPS. Statistical methods are also being called upon to assess quality variations as a function of broad organizational characteristics of health care delivery, such as the comparative quality associated with different types of hospitals (e.g., teaching versus nonteaching, hospitals with high volume for certain surgical procedures versus those with low volume); different reimbursement and practice organization arrangements (HMOs versus fee-for-service); different triage and referral arrangements (e.g., regionalization of trauma and emergency care); different types of physicians (specialists versus generalists, board-certified versus noncertified, foreign medical graduates versus U.S. graduates), and so forth.

Given their widespread and growing use, the validity of these statistical approaches in relation to case review is thus of much concern. This topic is, in fact, the subject of a three-year study currently being conducted by the Rand Corporation to determine whether "nonintrusive measures" such as mortality and hospital readmissions which can be easily obtained from secondary data sources are systematically related to process errors found through review of individual medical records.[10]

The Model for Statistical Evaluations of Quality

When discussing quality assessment, few people mention the large body of controlled clinical research that has been performed in recent years. This oversight is ironic because this research is the ultimate source of much information needed to develop and improve standards of care. The classic example of controlled clinical research is the controlled clinical trial in which patients are randomly assigned to alternative treatments. This research includes the extensive testing of pharmacological agents as well as the evaluation of the therapeutic efficacy of inverventions as diverse as extracranial-intracranial bypass to reduce the risk of strokes and early hospital discharge in uncomplicated myocardial infarction.[11,12] The results of these trials are often published in our major medical journals.

The results of this research are also frequently summarized by professional organizations and by expert panels convened by such organizations as the Congressional Office of Technology Assessment and the National Institutes of Health to formulate recommendations on new technologies or other treatment protocols.[13]

The results of these studies become the basis for the development of future process criteria. For example, controlled clinical research of recent years has resulted in a specific protocol to be followed in ruling out acute myocardial infarction. This protocol has become the basis for criteria used by some PROs in their assessment, through record review, of the quality of care in myocardial infarction.

Thus, controlled clinical research is at root a quality quantification tool. It is, perhaps, the definitive quality assessment tool since it provides a rigorous and systematic test of the outcome of a medical or surgical intervention. The act of random assignment of patients to treatments effectively controls for other factors which could be responsible for the outcome. Controlled clinical study has not been used to measure the performance of individual hospitals or physicians, although in theory it could be. In general, it has also not been used to assess structural aspects of health care delivery, such as the reimbursement method or delivery mode. Among the notable exceptions to this assertion is the Rand health insurance experiment, which, along with several similar studies, used random assignment to compare patient outcomes across different financing and reimbursement mechanisms.[14]

The disadvantages of controlled clinical research include the fact that it is very expensive to perform and is generally confined to the evaluation of new technologies and treatments or new applications of existing treatments. It cannot be used to assess most established treatments because it would preempt patient and physician freedom of choice. Additionally, once a therapy is widely accepted, ethical issues emerge which generally preclude experimentation and the random assignment of patients to conditions which are thought to be less efficacious. As a result, examination of many interventions must be done with naturally occurring data, that is, with nonexperimental designs.

Once the element of random assignment is eliminated from clinical research, the difficulty of interpretation increases dramatically, since the results may be due to a host of factors other than the intervention being tested. Good clinical research need not necessarily be confined to experimentally controlled studies, however. It may be performed through the use of statistical modeling. The two methods, controlled studies and statisical modeling, are compared by Krakauer as follows:

> The information gathered through modeling when applied to observational studies bears a marked resemblance to that obtained in randomized controlled trials. The purpose of such trials is to assess the impact of a risk factor or therapeutic intervention by comparing outcomes in a population subjected to the risk factor or intervention with outcomes in a population not subjected to this risk factor or intervention, but otherwise identical. Randomization [is the attempt to assure this identity in a clinical trial]. In modeling, the identity is achieved by a mathematical manipulation.[15]

There is thus a large body of clinical research which, although nonexperimental, still achieves high levels of rigor through sophisticated statistical control based on epidemiological models. The well-documented relationship between smoking and lung cancer is one example. Others include the Framingham Study of risk factors associated with heart disease, studies of the sociodemographic risk factors associated with premature birth, and a recent study of the relationship between hip fracture and use of estrogen in postmenopausal women.[16-18]

The statistical modeling approach is increasingly of interest in evaluating the impact not only of clinical interventions but also of some of the broader organizational interventions previously mentioned. Blumberg has produced a comprehensive review of the methodologies used in these studies.[19] He has summarized the methods under the rubric, "Risk Adjusted Monitoring of Outcomes" (RAMO). These methods, as the name implies, are outcome-oriented and transfer the epidemiological framework from clinical research to investigation through the use of administrative data. The most widely used methods in such RAMO studies involve patient classification and indirect standardization. Patients are first classified into risk-homogeneous categories based on their characteristics at the time of the intervention. Outcome rates are then calculated by patient category using data from a referent or baseline group of individuals who either received a different intervention or received no intervention at all. These rates are applied to the study group by patient category to obtain an expected outcome rate for that group in the absence of the intervention. If actual outcomes for the study group are better than the expected outcomes, the result can be attributed to greater efficacy (or better quality) of the treatment intervention. If outcomes are poorer than expected, this can be attributed to decreased efficacy (or poor quality).

An example of the application of RAMO methods to the assessment of quality is the current interest in evaluation of hospital care by the examination of mortality rates for different classes of patients. In such studies, admission to various hospitals is the treatment intervention being compared, and mortality is the outcome. How do these studies differ from the clinical research model on which they are based? The major difference is not so much in the methods used, but in the variables measured. Clinical research, whether experimental or nonexperimental, has tailored data collection efforts which produce measurements sufficiently refined to permit adequate statistical control of confounding factors. The mortality and readmission studies differ in that their data sources are not individually tailored to the question at hand. Rather, these studies draw upon the vast pool of administrative data that has been developed by the major payers over the past decade. These data, which were developed for the purpose of reimbursing providers and not for performing clinical evaluations, do not as yet incorporate the refined measures needed to evaluate outcomes optimally or to control adequately for patient risk factors (severity of illness). The requirements in these two areas are discussed below.

What Is An Outcome?

Clinical measures

The measures of outcome used in statistically oriented outcome assessment are very similar to those described previously for generic screening--illustrating the close relationship of the two approaches. The major difference is that statistical assessments of outcome, although they tend to concentrate on the compilation of statistics of adverse events, are not limited to such events. They can just as easily use measures of health outcomes that are better than expected.

The measures chosen as indicators vary with the unit of analysis; i.e., whether one is examining the outcomes for the entire society, a self-contained health system within that society, specific hospitals or individual practitioners. Outcome measures such as general health status, life expectancy, and deaths due to lung cancer can be used to measure societal factors external to the health delivery system, such as the adequacy of nutrition and living conditions, prevalence of good health practices and national commitment to minimizing exposure to toxic substances. Other measures may more narrowly assess the adequacy of a society's health delivery system, including not only its hospital system but its ambulatory and preventive care systems, its epidemiological monitoring systems, and its public health programs. A high incidence of low-birth weight infants, infectious diseases that are preventable through immunization programs, uncontrolled hypertension, deaths from cervical cancers, and late-stage admissions to hospitals all may indicate a health system that is functioning poorly. Since an HMO is a self-contained health system controlling all the health services delivered to its enrollees, many of these measures are pertinent to evaluating care delivered by these plans. (See Chapters 9 and 10.)

A third category of outcome measures specifically reflects the quality of care provided in hospital settings. This category includes discharge mortality, surgical mortality, and mortality occurring in a given time period following admission or discharge. It also includes various measures of morbidity (with or without permanent disability) caused by complications, misadventures of care, or by failure to provide needed care.

Utilization as a proxy for outcome

All the above are clinical measures reflecting actual patient health outcomes. Previously, we discussed the use of utilization measures as an indicator of quality, as in comparing, for example, surgical rates or immunization rates across different populations or time periods. As discussed, the utility of utilization measures depends on how well the utilization standards have been validated.

In addition to the ways previously discussed that utilization measures can complicate the analysis of quality, there is yet another. Utilization measures are frequently used as a proxy for outcome, based on the assumption that poor quality of care resulting in an adverse outcome in turn results in increased use of health services. Such measures may include unplanned return to the operating room, transfer to an ICU, increased length of stay, readmission, or increased use of subacute care and rehabilitative services.

Problems similar to those discussed previously arise in the use of these measures of utilization as a proxy for outcome. It has been widely established that the provision of most health services is not solely a function of clinical status, but depends also upon treatment philosophy, financial incentives, and the availability of alternate treatments. When such factors are operating, the provision of care cannot necessarily be taken as a measure of outcome. As an example, consider the interest following the introduction of PPS in the study of hospital readmissions as a measure of quality of care. An increase in readmissions may be expected to occur if patients were discharged prematurely and subsequently required readmission for problems which should have been resolved in the first stay. Readmissions may also occur, however, because under PPS the payment to hospitals is on a per-stay basis and there is thus an incentive to split care that may previously have been provided in a single hospital stay into two stays (e.g., to perform the preoperative work-up, discharge the patient, and then readmit the patient for the procedure itself). In any examination of readmission rates, the first type of behavior which represents a true quality problem would be confounded with the second type of behavior which is a treatment decision influenced by financial incentives.

Thus, in general, utilization should be used as a proxy measure for outcome only under limited circumstances. It is most appropriate when the service under consideration is not discretionary and is highly determined by clinical need. Unplanned return to the operating room is one such measure.

Issues In the Use of Mortality To Measure Quality

Clinical measures of outcome; e.g., morbidity and disability, are very often difficult to obtain without special data collection efforts. Morbidity is difficult to measure accurately because the coding of complications in existing data bases is largely unreliable. The presence of disability is similarly almost impossible to ascertain from such data bases. As a result, current efforts to assess outcomes have focused on mortality because it is the most easily measured

51

event and is also the most deleterious outcome. The use of mortality as a measure of outcome is likely to become increasingly prominent, as witnessed by its incorporation into the objectives of the PROs and HCFA's two releases of hospital-specific mortality data.

Whereas mortality would appear a fairly simple and straight-forward outcome measure, the interpretation of studies using mortality as a measure of quality is by no means simple or straightforward. The problems noted with these studies are many and provide a flavor of the kinds of measurement and statistical problems facing studies of outcomes using administrative data. (See Chapter 1; for an alternative viewpoint, see Chapter 7.)

One problem with the current mortality studies relates to the time period within which mortality is measured. HCFA's 1985 data on mortality by hospital used discharge mortality as its outcome measure; that is, death which occurs during the inpatient stay, rather than following discharge. These statistics have shown that, for the Medicare population, California hospitals have a discharge mortality of 5.9 percent, whereas New York hospitals have a discharge mortality of 8.6 percent. New York hospitals, however, have a substantially greater length of stay than California hospitals which creates a greater opportunity for death to occur while patients are in the hospital. If the outcome measure is redefined as mortality occurring within 30 days of admission regardless of whether in the hospital or not, the differences between California and New York disappear. Mortality in a given time period following admission, rather than discharge mortality, is thus a more appropriate indicator of hospital quality.[20]

There are other statistical problems associated with the use of mortality as an outcome measure. Reviewing the HCFA mortality analysis, Blumberg summarized a number of them.[21] First, an examination of the residuals of the HCFA statistical model indicates that the model is biased ("compressed") and therein both underestimates expected mortality at the high end of the distribution and overestimates it at the low end. In nontechnical terms, the implication of this bias is that, when actual outcomes are compared with expected outcomes, high-risk hospitals appear to do much worse than expected and low-risk hospitals much better. Another type of bias in HCFA's model is the fact that the t-test statistic used to assess the significance of deviation from expected mortality is not sensitive in comparing actual with predicted death when the expected number of deaths is very low. As a result, small hospitals appear to have a higher rate of excess deaths than large hospitals.

Concerns have also been expressed about the use of mortality as an outcome measure in surgical volume studies. Beginning with the Stanford Institutional Differences Study in 1974, researchers have consistently found that hospitals performing a higher volume of a given procedure tend to have lower mortality rates for that procedure.[22-25] The utility of this finding in identifying poor-quality providers is unclear, however. Luft notes that although this relationship is strong when hospitals are aggregated by type in the analysis, it cannot be used to identify individual hospitals with high death rates reliably, because of the small cell sizes which result when data are subdivided by both hospital and type of procedure.[26] The resulting possibility is that the observed negative outcomes are a statistical artifact of these small samples and are not caused by poor care.

The most serious and vociferously expressed concerns about mortality studies entail the adequacy of statistical control of other patient factors affecting outcome. The concerns are not confined to mortality studies, but relate to any statistical examination of outcomes. To be meaningful, statistical assessments of outcome must adequately control for patient risk factors. Prominent among these risk factors is the severity of the patient's illness.

Controlling For Patient Severity

Systems that measure the severity of a patient's illness provide a means to control patient-specific, disease-related factors; i.e., the degree of sickness of a patient, so that observed differences in outcome data across different populations of patients may be meaningfully used to infer differences in the quality of care rendered. (See Chapter 3.) Although promoted as quality assessment tools, these systems are not in themselves quality tools, and they have uses which go beyond the measurement of quality. In fact, they are required for adequate interpretation of almost all analyses of nonexperimental patient-level data. For instance, sicker patients require more resources in their treatment and are therefore more costly to treat. Severity measures are thus needed in any examination of resource consumption. For example, a hospital might be interested in measuring the severity of illness of its patients to ascertain whether physicians whose patients have longer lengths of stay and more expensive treatment patterns have truly sicker patients or are merely more inefficient in managing care. Similarly, a state reimbursement agency may wish to ascertain whether higher payments to certain hospitals (e.g., teaching hospitals) are justified on the grounds that they have sicker patients. Today, the use of severity systems and related patient classification systems is commonplace. The major issue with these systems is how to improve them using more refined measures of patient severity.

In addition to being more costly to treat, sicker patients also have poorer outcomes. For that reason, any comparison of health outcomes between settings requires that the severity of illness of the patients in the two settings be measured and that the observed outcomes be adjusted to control for the differences in severity. Only when this adjustment is made can one be confident that the difference in the observed outcomes is caused by the quality of care received, as opposed to differing levels of severity of illness.

The importance of considering patient severity when analyzing differences in outcomes across settings is illustrated in a recent study from the Rand Corporation.[27] In this study, hospitals with higher than expected mortality rates were compared with those with lower than expected rates. In a review of the medical records of patients discharged dead from these hospitals, precise measures of illness severity abstracted from the medical record accounted almost entirely for the difference in mortality between the two sets of hospitals. There was, however, on the basis of physician chart review, a small but statistically significantly higher percentage of deaths judged to be preventable in the high-mortality hospitals than in the lower-mortality hospitals.

There are currently five systems for measuring severity in varying degrees of general use. Each of these has undergone, and is continuing to undergo, extensive development and testing, largely with funding from the federal government. These are:

■ Medical Illness Severity Groups (MedisGroups), developed by Charles Jacobs, J.D., and Alan Brewster, M.D., of Mediqual Systems, Inc.[28];

■ Disease Staging, developed by Joseph Gonnella, M.D., and colleagues, of Thomas Jefferson University in conjunction with researchers at SysteMetrics/McGraw-Hill[29,30]

■ Patient Management Categories (PMCs), developed by Wanda Young, Ph.D., at Blue Cross of Pennsylvania[31];

■ Computerized Severity Index (CSI), developed by Susan Horn, Ph.D., and researchers at Johns Hopkins University and Health Systems, Inc.[32]; and

■ Acute Physiological and Chronic Health Evaluation (APACHE), developed by William Knaus, M.D., and colleagues at the George Washington University.[33]

In general, these severity systems rely primarily on clinical information concerning the patient's condition to measure severity. Some severity systems also consider information on treatment decisions in determining severity. PMCs, like DRGs, consider whether a major surgical procedure is performed in assigning patients to categories. Some systems use such treatment decisions, such as placement in an ICU, as an indicator of severity. CSI additionally bases severity determinations on the rate of response to therapy, on the assumption that more severely ill patients will take longer to recover.

The ways in which these systems characterize severity are also diverse. Certain systems (MedisGroups, APACHE, and CSI) assign a single severity score to a case based on a weighted sum of the various severity factors described above. The score assigned is independent of the principal diagnosis. PMCs, like DRGs, classify patients into distinct categories and thus more closely resemble a case-mix system than a severity system per se. (A case-mix system can be used just as well as a severity system to perform risk adjustments, as long as the case-mix categories are predictive of outcomes.) Disease Staging is diagnosis-specific and assigns an ordinal severity score to a given patient based on the patient's stage of illness in the natural continuum of disease progression. Two of the severity systems, Disease Staging and APACHE, are described further in Chapters 3 and 4, respectively.

An in-depth discussion of the merits of each of these five systems is beyond the scope of this chapter. Each continues to be refined by its developers, and extensive research on the strengths, weaknesses, and potential applications of these systems is under way. One area under particular scrutiny is their use as a refinement of the DRG system.[34] Development of an easily applied tool which can characterize the important clinical dimensions of every hospitalized patient is an ambitious task, and there is a great deal of work still to be done before we accomplish this goal. In this effort to refine the above measurement systems, the particular requirements of quality measurement, as opposed to other uses for these systems, should be kept firmly in mind. The requirements for quality measurement are more restrictive than other applications.

One such requirement has been noted by Blumberg (see note 18). To serve its function of risk adjusting outcome data, the severity measure must do just that; i.e., it should measure risk at the outset of the intervention and not measure other clinical events which occur in the hospital and may be the adverse result of treatment. While this is a straightforward concept, most administrative data systems do not allow for the differentiation of comorbid conditions and other factors present on admission from complications that occur after admission. This effectively eliminates DRGs from consideration as a true risk adjustment system since DRGs disregard the distinction between comorbid conditions and complications. A similar argument pertains to the use of the length of time required for a patient to respond to treatment as a measure of severity, since the patient's response will be a function not only of the severity of illness but also of the quality of care received.

Another requirement for risk adjusting severity systems is that they should be pure measures of patient clinical factors and should not incorporate treatment decisions in their algorithms. It is true that for patients who are more severely ill, the intervention will often be more intense, resulting, for example, in placement in an ICU, in more invasive interventions, or in longer lengths of stay. However, given the wide variety of practice styles, such process items, as noted previously, are not unambiguous measures of either patient risk or patient outcome. While they may be appropriately used to measure case mix for reimbursement purposes, they do not have the clinical purity needed in the area of quality assessment.

Another consideration relating to the evaluation of severity systems is the trade off between parsimony and precision. While it is appealing to have a system based on a minimal set of key indicators, it is questionable that such a system validly predicts risk factors for all conditions. APACHE, for example, uses 12 physiologic measures (e.g., heart rate, blood pressure, serum potassium levels, serum pH, etc.) to characterize severity. (See Chapter 4.) APACHE has been applied quite successfully to analysis of critically ill patients, patients who despite the underlying cause of their disease have deteriorated to the point that there is substantial compromise of vital organ systems.[35] Such physiologic factors are not, however, as predictive of outcome for patients not close to death. For cancer patients, factors such as size of tumor mass and the extent of metastases, for example, are far better variables for characterizing disease severity and predicting outcome. Also, for cancer patients, research by Garber et al. suggests that, in addition to clinical factors such as stage of disease, one must consider the reason for admission (diagnostic, restorative, palliative, or terminal care) to predict accurately outcome in these cases.[36]

Perhaps the biggest deficiencies in the various severity systems are not related so much to the systems themselves, but to the present form of the administrative data they are designed to use. Three of the systems (MedisGroups, APACHE, and CSI) require special data collection such as medical record abstraction. PMCs are used only with computerized patient abstract data. Disease Staging has both a clinical version for primary data collection and an automated version for use with patient abstract or billing data. (See Chapter 3.) The computerized version is necessarily an imperfect rendition of the clinical version, but one which is presumably correctable with better automated data.

One problem with automated data in their present form is that they are capable of reflecting only those differences in severity which can be expressed in diagnostic labeling. Differences which depend upon specification of laboratory values or radiological findings, for example, require specially abstracted data. If widescale quality assessment using administrative data is to become a reality, there will necessarily have to be improvements in administrative data collection to accommodate them. In addition, if the precision inherent in the data obtained through primary data collection is desired on a wide-scale basis, the costs of this data collection will have to be realistically factored into hospital payment systems.

CONCLUSION

Whether PPS has had as deleterious effect on quality as feared, it has focused attention on quality of care. The ferment in the quality area is taking many forms. It has resulted in widespread use and interest in generic screens by the PROs. (See Chapter 6.) Similarly, the examination of the quality of care provided Medicare beneficiaries in capitated plans has focused attention on system-wide measures of quality, not just in that provided in hospitals. (See Chapter 9.) Most of all, there has been widespread interest in assessing broad measures of system performance through use of, and upgrading of, routinely collected administrative data.

Figure 5 summarizes the various approaches to quality measurement, presenting both their advantages and disadvantages. Each of these approaches has something unique to offer and all may be needed in a complete quality monitoring system. It is not difficult to predict that methods of quality quantification will become increasingly more sophisticated. Advances that might be expected in the near future include:

- changes in data systems themselves to capture more sophisticated predictors of patient severity factors;

- changes in data systems to capture more sophisticated measures of patient outcome;

- continued enhancement, refinement, and validation of patient severity systems;

- continued refinement of statistical approaches to measuring quality to eliminate unintended biases; and

- expansion of quality monitoring beyond the inpatient setting to ambulatory care, long-term care, and total system performance.

Figure 1. The two methodologic approaches to quality assessment.

Methodological Approach	Characteristics
I. Case Review	Direct measurement through comparison with clinical norms
	Assigns a judgment to a single case
	Process-oriented
	Manual application
	High cost per case
	Reliability may be an issue
II. Statistical Assessment	Indirect measurement through comparison with norms
	Quantifies quality only in the aggregate
	Outcome-oriented
	Computerized
	Low cost per case
	Validity may be an issue

Figure 2. Specific varieties of quality assessment methods.

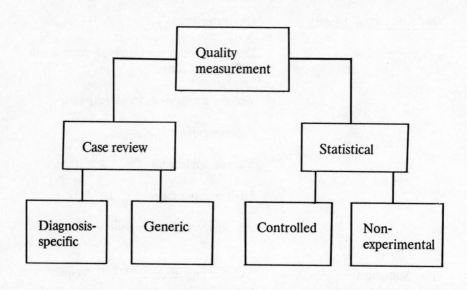

Figure 3. Example "list" criteria for appropriateness of clinical management in the emergency room of cardiac patients who are not experiencing a cardiopulmonary arrest.*

Management of cardiac patients in the ER prior to transfer to an intensive care unit is appropriate if:

1. Patient is placed on cardiac monitor with at least one printout strip.

2. Printout strip is interpreted correctly.

3. Complete vital signs evaluation is repeated at least every 30 minutes.

4. Intravenous access is established by drip or lock.

5. Oxygen is administered at 21/min. or more.

6. Pain medication is appropriate in dose, route, and frequency of administration.

7. Family or significant other is notified.

8. Attending physician is notified.

9. Patient is transferred to CCU with monitor/defibrillator.

*Taken from *The Monitoring Sourcebook*, Physician Practice Monitors, Vol. 3 (Chicago: Care Communications, Inc., 1986).

Figure 4. The six HCFA generic screens.

1. Adequacy of discharge planning

    ■ No documented plan for appropriate follow-up care or discharge planning as necessary, with consideration of physical, emotional, and mental status/needs at the time of discharge.

2. Medical stability of the patient at discharge

    ■ BP on day before or day of discharge: systolic--less than 85 or greater than 180; diastolic--less than 50 or greater than 110
    ■ Temperature on day before or day of discharge greater than 101 degrees oral (rectal 102 degrees)
    ■ Pulse less than 50 (or 45 if the patient is on a beta blocker) or greater than 120 within 24 hours of discharge
    ■ Abnormal results of diagnostic services which are not addressed or explained in the medical record
    ■ IV fluids or drugs on the day of discharge (excludes KVOs, antibiotics, chemotherapy, or total parenteral nutrition)
    ■ Purulent or bloody drainage of postoperative wound within 24 hours prior to discharge

3. Deaths

    ■ During or following elective surgery
    ■ Following return to intensive care unit, coronary care or special care unit within 24 hours of being transferred out
    ■ Other unexpected death

4. Nosocomial infections

    ■ Temperature increase of more than 2 degrees more than 72 hours from admission
    ■ Indication of infection following an invasive procedure (e.g., suctioning, catheter insertion, tube feedings, surgery, etc.)

5. Unscheduled return to surgery within same admission for same condition as previous surgery or to correct operative problem (exclude "staged" procedures)

6. Trauma suffered in the hospital

   ■ Unplanned removal or repair of a normal organ (i.e., removal or repair not addressed in operative consent)
   ■ Fall with injury or untoward effect (including but not limited to fracture, dislocation, concussion, laceration, etc.)
   ■ Life-threatening complications of anesthesia
   ■ Life-threatening transfusion error or reaction
   ■ Hospital-acquired decubitus ulcer
   ■ Care resulting in serious or life-threatening complications, not related to admitting signs and symptoms, including but not limited to the neurological, endocrine, cardiovascular, renal, or respiratory body systems (e.g., resulting in dialysis, unplanned transfer to special care unit, lengthened hospital stay)
   ■ Major adverse drug reaction or medication error with serious potential for harm or resulting in special measures to correct (e.g., intubation, cardio-pulmonary resuscitation, gastric lavage) including but not limited to the following:
       ■ Incorrect antibiotic ordered by the physician (e.g., inconsistent with diagnostic studies or the patient's history of drug allergy)
       ■ No diagnostic studies to confirm which drug is correct to administer (e.g., C&S)
       ■ Serum drug levels not performed as needed
       ■ Diagnostic studies or other measures for side effects not performed as needed (e.g., BUN, creatinine, intake and output)

Figure 5. Comparison of quality assessment methods.

	Diagnosis-Specific Case Review	Generic Case Review	Controlled Clinical Trials	Nonexperimental Outcome Analysis
Advantages	Detects problems with potential as well as actual harm Measures the whole spectrum of quality Generally relies on explicit criteria	Focuses on worst outcomes Efficient for widescale monitoring	Most definitive method of linking process/treatments with outcome True outcome orientation	Efficient for widescale monitoring Detects patterns too subtle to identify through record review of a small number of cases
Disadvantages	High cost per case Narrow focus Difficult to quantify impact of process errors Some subjective clinical judgment required	Neglects events with potential rather than actual harm Requires subjective clinical evaluation Attribution of error not always possible through record review	High cost per case Interferes with freedom of choice	Requires good measures of outcome, severity of illness and other risk factors for definitive results
Uses	Focused review Provides quality assurance Training and behavior change	Provider quality assurance Ongoing monitoring of sample of cases Training and behavior change	Testing of new treatment interventions or new applications of old treatments	Widescale monitoring Evaluates organizational characteristics of health care delivery and existing standards of practice

NOTES

1.   J. Wennberg, "Which Rate is Right?," *New England Journal of Medicine,* 314(1986): 310-311.

2.   N.J. Merrick, et al., "Use of Carotid Endarterectomy in Five California Veterans Administration Medical Centers," *Journal of the American Medical Association,* 256(1986): 2531-2535.

3.   J. Wennberg, "Setting Outcome-Based Standards for Carotid Endarterectomy," *Journal of the American Medical Association,* 256(1986): 2566.

4.   S. Greenfield, et al., "Comparison of a Criteria Map to a Criteria List in Quality of Care Assessment for Patients with Chest Pain: The Relation of Each to Outcome," *Medical Care,* 19(1981): 255-271.

5.   D.M. Kessner, C.E. Kalk, and J. Singer, "Assessing Health Quality: The Case for Tracers," *New England Journal of Medicine,* 288(1973): 189-194.

6.   J.W. Craddick and B.S. Bader, *Medical Management Analysis: A Systematic Approach to Quality Assurance and Risk Management: Volume 1, An Introduction* (Auburn, CA: Joyce W. Craddick, 1983).

7.   D. Rutstein, et al., "Measuring the Quality of Medical Care: A Clinical Method," *New England Journal of Medicine,* 294(1976): 582-588.

8.   R.G. Petersdorf, et al., *Harrison's Principles of Internal Medicine* (New York: McGraw-Hill, 1983).

9.   Joint Commission on Accreditation of Healthcare Organizations, Agenda for Change, Chicago, IL, November 1986.

10. *Status Report: Research and Demonstrations in Health Care Financing* (Baltimore, MD: Health Care Financing Administration, January 1986).

11. J.C. Grotta, "Current Medical and Surgical Therapy for Cerebro-vascular Disease," *New England Journal of Medicine,* 317(1987): 1505-1516.

12. G. Ahlmark, et al., "A Controlled Study of Early Discharge after Uncomplicated Mycardial Infarction," *Acta Medica Scandinavia,* 206(1979): 87-91.

13. S. Perry, "The NIH Consensus Development Program: A Decade Later," *New England Journal of Medicine,* 317(1987): 485-488.

14. J.E. Ware, et al., "Comparison of Health Outcomes at a Health Maintenance Organization with Those of Fee for Service Care," *The Lancet,* I(1986): 1017-1022.

15. H. Krakauer, *Modeling in the Analysis of Survival Data* (Bethesda MD: National Institute of Allergy and Infectious Diseases, National Institutes of Health, no date).

16. T.R. Dawber, *The Framingham Study: The Epidemiology of Atherosclerotic Disease* (Cambridge, MA: Harvard University Press, 1980).

17. D.P. Kiel, et al., "Hip Fracture and the Use of Estrogens in Postmenopausal Women," *New England Journal of Medicine,* 317(1987): 1169-1174.

18. E. Lieberman, et al., "Risk Factors Accounting for Racial Differences in the Rate of Premature Births," *New England Journal of Medicine,* 317(1987): 743-748.

19. M.S. Blumberg, "Risk Adjusting Health Care Outcomes: A Methodologic Review," *Medical Care Review,* 43(1986): 351-393.

20. P. Eggers, Unpublished data from the Health Care Financing Administration, personal communication, 1988.

Chapter 3

Severity of Illness in the Assessment of Quality: Disease Staging

Joseph S. Gonnella, M.D., and Daniel Z. Louis

Effective quality assurance and utilization review functions require the identification of groups of patients whose medical needs and prognoses are similar.[1,2] Ideally, they require a system for such patient identification. Such a system would permit analysis of whether patients with "similar illnesses" were managed in similar ways and also provide a means for comparing outcomes of care among providers and institutions. The challenge, of course, is how to develop such a system; specifically how to define and measure similar illnesses.[3] A number of questions should be asked, including the following:

1). How can/should similarity in disease be defined? What are the essential disease characteristics which allow different diseases to be classified in common categories and allow cases with a given disease to be classified by severity?

2). How much similarity, homogeneity, or specificity is necessary for a classification system?

3). When in the treatment process should definitions of similarity be applied?

4). What factors, other than biological similarity of disease will, or should, influence the utilization of health care resources and expected patient outcomes?

DEFINITION OF DISEASE

Health problems--symptoms, physical abnormalities, and pathological findings--are often classified, coded, and analyzed as if they were equivalent to disease.[4] As manifestations of physiological/psychological functions, identification of these problems is an important part of the diagnostic process. Classification of patients by their health problems, is not sufficient for analysis of quality of care, appropriate treatment, or expected outcomes. In addition to pathophysiology, etiology and severity are essential elements of a disease.

Unfortunately, many diagnostic labels traditionally used by medical professionals and most diagnositc rubrics used in the various coding systems (e.g., *The International Classification of Diseases: Clinical Modification*[5]) do not provide information on these elements. Thus, with these systems, patients are often classified into inappropriate groups. As a result, the overall severity of disease for any group of patients cannot be assessed, and comparison between various treatments, providers, and institutions cannot be appropriately made.

Diseases should be distinguished from health problems. A diagnosis should, whenever possible, provide the information necessary to document the four elements required to define a specific disease. These four elements of a diagnosis--the location of the problem, the etiologies of the problem, the pathophysiological change characteristic of the problem, and the severity of the problem--are displayed in Figure 1.

The location of the problem should be specified. Shown in Figure 1 as an organ system, the location of the problem should be identified as specifically as possible in terms of the involvement of organ systems, organs, or parts of organs. Thus, in a patient with coronary artery disease, the specific arteries involved should be specified.

The etiological factor or set of factors responsible for the pathophysiological changes must be identified whenever possible. Neither pneumonia nor bronchial pneumonia meets this criterion. The specific bacterium or virus causing the pneumonia should be documented. A health problem such as congestive heart failure (CHF) that may result from a variety of causes is not a disease, even though CHF may be coded as such and may be the principal diagnosis now appearing on many medical records and discharge abstracts.

A disease definition should specify the characteristic pathophysiological change in the involved organ or organ system. A diagnosis of "peptic ulcer" provides inadequate information; upper gastrointestinal tract bleeding secondary to peptic ulcer provides more specific information. Severity of the pathophysiological changes must also be given. This can be done by specifying the stage of the disease. For instance, pneumococcal pneumonia with septicemia is a disease at a very different severity level, and with very different expected outcome, than pneumococcal pneumonia without complications.

It is important to stress the need to identify all four elements in order to completely specify a disease and allow meaningful comparisons among providers or institutions. A number of severity measurement systems (e.g., APACHE II, MedisGroups) focus on laboratory data but ignore the etiology of the problem.[6] This type of approach limits the utility of such systems. For example, knowing that a patient has a hemoglobin of six may be sufficient to determine the need for hospital admission. However, one would need also to know the cause of the anemia (e.g., nutritional, blood loss secondary to peptic ulcer, cancer of the colon, uterine fibroma, bone marrow failure due to leukemia or other causes) in order to evaluate prognosis or the quality of care provided.

DISEASE STAGING

In staging, diseases are divided into categories of increasing levels of severity: Stage 1, conditions with no complications or problems of minimal severity; Stage 2, problems limited to an organ or system, significantly increased risk of complications over Stage 1; Stage 3, multiple site involvement, generalized systemic involvement, poor prognosis; Stage 4, death.[7,8,9]

Staging does not depend on utilization patterns or on expected response to therapy to assess severity. It is based on a conceptual model of the disease process itself rather than on the relative efficacy of medical technology. Developed and tested over a period of fifteen years, staging criteria are now available for approximately 400 diseases.[10] These include the major diseases in etiology and body system class and represent the vast majority of admissions to a typical short-term hospital.

Samples of staging criteria for appendicitis and coronary artery disease are shown in Table 1 and Table 2. In addition to the descriptions of the disease stages, each criteria set includes the specification of the physical findings, laboratory data, pathology and X-ray reports necessary for patient classification.

71

The staging criteria can be applied directly if medical records are available. While this is not a problem for many quality assurance and utilization review activities, it may be too costly and time consuming for large scale research or utilization analysis projects. In order to apply staging to large discharge abstract data bases, the staging criteria have been translated into "coded" staging criteria using the ICD-9 CM coding system. Each statement in the staging criteria sets is represented by all possible codes or combinations of codes that reflect the conditions in that statement as accurately as the coding system will allow.[11,12] Therefore, staging can be applied directly to medical records data or existing coded data bases, or by using a combination of the two types of information.

APPLICATION TO QUALITY ASSURANCE AND UTILIZATION REVIEW

As a clinically based patient classification system that captures the critical dimension of severity of illness, disease staging can be used as a part of many quality assurance and utilization review activities.[13,14] For example, the admission review process is largely one of timing in the use of health care services; that is, the review determines whether inpatient health care services might have been used more appropriately at an earlier or later time in the disease process. There are four possibilities with regard to the timing of a hospital admission:

1). The patient had no medical indications for either diagnostic or therapeutic intervention requiring acute care hospitalization.

2). The patient was admitted too early (i.e., the diagnostic or therapeutic intervention could have taken place in an ambulatory setting).

3). The patient's hospitalization was appropriate.

4). The patient was admitted too late (i.e., a complication exists which might have been prevented had hospitalization occurred earlier in the disease process).

The staging criteria can be used to systematize the decision-making process necessary to determine whether or not a patient is "sick enough" to justify admission to an acute care institution. For each disease, a threshold stage can be identified at which the admission will be considered appropriate. A patient with a diagnosis of Stage 1 appendicitis or unstable angina pectoris (Stage 2.5, coronary artery disease) is hospitalized appropriately. Conversely, the admission of a patient with Stage 1 hypertension or diabetes mellitus should be questioned unless the patient has other disabilities which justify hospitalization.[15]

Staging can be used to assure effective and efficient review of hospital services. Length of stay norms should be adjusted to account for stage of illness. One would expect a longer length of stay with more intense care provided for a Stage 2 appendicitis patient with a retroperitoneal abscess than for a Stage 1 patient with simple appendicitis.[16] Patients falling outside expected margins, (for example, patients with especially long lengths of stay given their stage of illness) represent potential quality-of-care problems. These differences in utilization patterns as a function of the stage of illness can be built into a hospital's quality assurance and utilization review activities.

Using patients with diabetes mellitus, as an example, some of the applications of disease staging to quality assurance activities can be outlined.[17,18] The first step for a hospital (or health maintenance organization or employer) would be to identify all patients with a diagnosis of diabetes mellitus and classify them by stage of illness. Patients with advanced-stage diabetes mellitus represent potential quality of care problems and require further analysis.

The first questions to be addressed are: When in the process of care did the complication(s) occur? Did it occur before the patient sought medical care or after the patient was seen by a physician (before or after hospitalization)?

The answer to these questions identifies the area requiring further audit. If the complication did not occur until after hospitalization, was the cause delayed diagnosis and/or treatment, (e.g., the result of physician or laboratory error)? If it was institutional delay, what was the reason for it? If the complication occurred prior to the patient seeking care, was it the result of a lack of health facilities, ignorance, financial barriers, or simply a rapid onset of the disease? If the complication occurred while under the care of a physician, was it a result of physician error (e.g., misdiagnosis, delayed or inappropriate treatment), or lack of compliance with a recommended treatment regimen?

Table 3 displays the distribution of diabetes mellitus patients at one hospital by stage of illness. It is clear from this example that all patients with this diagnosis are not clinically homogeneous. The Stage 2 and Stage 3 patients have longer lengths of stay as well as more costly hospitalizations in terms of both duration of stay and per-diem cost.

Reviewing these data should give rise to a number of questions, including the following:

1). Was hospitalization required for the Stage 1 patients or could they have been treated in a less costly environment?

2). Could anything have been done to prevent the disease from progressing to Stage 2 or Stage 3? Was this progression a function of physician-related problems (e.g., late diagnosis/treatment), patient-related problems (e.g., poor compliance), financial or other barriers to care, or an unpreventable disease progression?

3). Are the hospital's review protocols designed to account for the differences in appropriate treatment patterns for these patients?

CONCLUSION

Effective quality assurance and utilization review functions require the identification of groups of patients whose medical needs are similar. Disease staging is such a clinically based patient classification system. Analysis of utilization patterns without the use of such a system can be misleading and result in serious consequences for the health care delivery system.

There are significant differences between hospitals in the proportions in the advanced stages. In many cases, the diagnosis related group (DRG) patient classification does not capture these differences.[19,20] Programs designed to reimburse hospitals or to identify "efficient" hospitals for negotiation of preferred-provider type arrangements must account for these differences or run the risk of misidentifying the efficient providers. It may, in the long run, also be counterproductive in their cost control efforts.

Even if no interhospital comparisons are being made, quality assurance or utilization review functions based on clinically hetero-geneous groups can result in misleading information. Assuming that all patients in a particular DRG or that all patients with congestive heart failure or pneumonia require similar treatment protocols or exhibit similar utilization patterns or mortality rates, is obviously not appropriate. For example, bacterial pneumonia patients treated at one hospital had an inpatient mortality rate of 7 percent. More thorough analysis of these data revealed mortality rates of 2 percent for those admitted at early stages of the disease and 28 percent for those admitted at later stages of the disease.

Disease staging can contribute significantly to the solution of these problems. An important characteristic of the staging approach is its emphasis on the medical meaningfulness of the criteria. While numerous analyses have demonstrated the strong relationship between staging and resource consumption, it is important to emphasize that no utilization data were used to develop the staging criteria.[21,22,23,24] This measure has an underlying conceptual structure in which only the clinically pertinent attributes of the patient's illness are employed in the classification system.

Disease staging is the most specific biological measure used to classify patients. Its four dimensions (etiology, organ involvement, pathophysiological change, and rank of complications) provide relevant clinical data to analyze prognosis, timeliness, and appropriateness of diagnostic and therapeutic interventions. Disease staging should be an integral part of systems developed for quality assurance or analysis of utilization of resources. It should not, however, be the sole variable.

In addition to the stage of the illness, other variables which should be included are: 1) presence of unrelated medical problems (e.g., presence and stage of diabetes mellitus in a patient hospitalized for appendicitis); 2) reason for admission (e.g., for diagnostic purposes only, for therapeutic purposes, for both diagnosis and therapy, for chemotherapy only, for observation only) and; 3) the use of surgical procedures or special units (e.g., intensive care units, coronary care units), if such use is justified by the needs of the patient. In addition--and ideally, as indicated in Chapter 1, the social support needs of the patient should be taken into account. This last variable will have an impact on timing of hospitalization and length of stay rather than on diagnostic or therapeutic intervention.

The use of resources depends not only on the clinical status of the patient, but also on the reason for admission and whether the latter is the first, or one of many, readmissions. For instance, a woman with Stage 3 cancer of the breast will consume more resources during the first hospitalization since at that time more diagnostic and therapeutic interventions will be used than on her third hospitalization when, for the same problem (Stage 3), it is likely that only chemotherapy or radiation therapy will be used.

In 1748, John Fothergill wrote a paper entitled "An Account of the Sore Throat with Ulcers," in which he reviewed the appropriate treatment for what was later called diphtheria.[25] In order to identify the appropriate treatment, Fothergill found it necessary to define four "periods" of the disease, since the treatment recommended for the first ("...vinegar in barley water, juice of pomegranate, syrup of roses...or a decoction of barley, red roses, liquorice and plantain...") would not be effective if the disease had advanced to "the second stage...wherein white sloughs begin to appear [where]...mild abstergents and antiputrescents, such as a decoction of lupins, beans, vetches, with honey of roses..." was necessary, or the fourth stage, in which case "...the fume of white amber thrown on live coals, and received into the mouth..." was advised.[26]

While Fothergill probably never dreamed of the advances in medicine over the last two centuries, and certainly never conceived of prospective payment systems, peer review organizations, or quality assurance committees, the principles he was following remain valid today. He recognized the need to define the stages of disease in order to specify appropriate treatment.

Disease is not a single static entity. One cannot evaluate appropriate treatment, the quality of care provided, or the expected outcome without first defining clinically homogeneous groups of patients. The disease staging approach to the definition and measurement of severity of illness provides a means for the definition of such groups.

Table 1

Staging Criteria

Appendicitis

Stage	Description
1.1	Appendicitis
2.1	Appendicitis with gross perforation leading to peritonitis or abscess in peritoneum or abscess in retroperitoneal space
2.2	Appendicitis with gross perforation leading to generalized peritonitis
2.3	Intestinal obstruction
2.4	Pylephebitis with or without liver abscess
3.1	Septicemia
3.2	Shock
4.0	Death

Table 2

Staging Criteria

Coronary artery diseases/acute myocardial infarction
(Atherosclerosis of coronary arteries, angina pectoris,
acute myocardial infarction, congestive heart failure
secondary to coronary artery disease)

Stage	Description
1.1	Angina pectoris--stable
2.1	Angina pectoris--progressing
2.2	Angina pectoris with abnormal cardiac findings
2.3	Angina pectoris with minimal evidence of congestive heart failure (CHF)
2.4	Angina pectoris with moderate evidence of congestive heart failure (CHF)
2.5	Angina pectoris--unstable or crescendo
2.6	Angina pectoris at rest
3.1	Acute myocardial infarction
3.2	Acute myocardial infarction and: heart block or supraventricular arrhythmmia or ventricular arrhythmia other than fibrillation or pericarditis

Table 2, continued

Staging Criteria

Stage	Description
3.3	Acute myocardial infarction and congestive heart failure (CHF)
3.4	Acute myocardial infarction and emboli to other organ(s)
3.5	Acute myocardial infarction and ventricular aneurysm
3.6	Acute myocardial infarction and: papillary muscle rupture or ventricular septal rupture
3.7	Acute myocardial infarction and cerebral vascular accident (CVA)
3.8	Acute myocardial infarction and: ventricular fibrillation or pulmonary edema or shock
3.9	Cardiac arrest
4.0	Death

Table 3

Distribution of Patients With Diabetes Mellitus From Sample Hospital by Stage of Illness

State	No. of	Percentage	Average length of stay	Average cost (1983 $)	Average cost per day
1	19	42.2	5.8	$2,341	$404
2	20	44.4	7.1	3,594	506
3	6	13.3	18.5	21,738	1,175
All	45	100.0	8.1	5,484	677

Figure 1. Elements of disease specification.

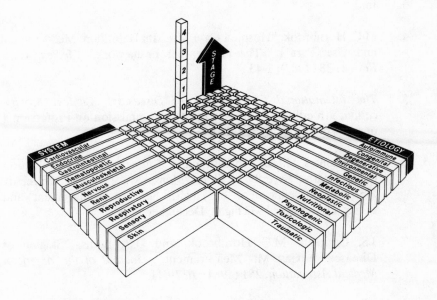

NOTES

1. J.S. Gonnella, "Patient Case Mix: Implications for Medical Educational and Hospital Costs," *Journal of Medical Education*, 56 (1981): 610-611.

2. J.S. Gonnella and C. Zeleznik, "Prospective Reimbursement Using the DRG Case Mix Classification System: A Medical Perspective," in: *Symposium on Contemporary Issues in Health Care* (Seattle, WA: Virginia Mason Medical Foundation, 1983).

3. Ibid.

4. M.C. Hornbrook, "Hospital Case Mix: Its Definition, Measurement and Use: Part I. The Conceptual Framework," *Medical Care Review*, 38 (1982): 1-43.

5. *The International Classification of Diseases: Clinical Modification*, 9th edition (Ann Arbor, MI: Commission on Professional and Hospital Activities, 1978).

6. J.W. Thomas, M.L.F. Ashcraft, and J. Zimmerman, "An Evaluation of Alternative Severity of Illness Measures for Use by University Hospitals" (Department of Health Services Management and Policy, University of Michigan, December 1986).

7. J.S. Gonnella, M.C. Hornbrook, and D.Z. Louis, "Staging of Disease: A Case-Mix Measurement," *Journal of the American Medical Association*, 251 (1984): 637-644.

8. J.S. Gonnella, D.Z. Louis, and J.J. McCord, "The Staging Concept --An Approach to the Assessment of Outcome of Ambulatory Care," *Medical Care*, 14 (1976): 13-21.

9. SysteMetrics, Inc., *Disease Staging: A Clinically Based Approach to Measurement of Disease Severity*, vols. 1 and 2, (final report, contract 233-78-3001) (Washington, DC: National Center for Health Services Research, 1983).

10. J.S. Gonnella, ed., *Disease Staging Clinical Criteria*, 3rd edition (Santa Barbara, CA: SysteMetrics/McGraw-Hill, 1986).

11. SysteMetrics, Inc., *Disease Staging: A Clinically Based Approach to Measurement of Disease Severity*, vol. 3, (final report, contract 233-78-3001) (Washington, DC: National Center for Health Services Research, 1983).

12. SysteMetrics, Inc., *Disease Staging: A Clinically Based Approach to Measurement of Disease Severity*, vol. 4, (final report, contract 233-78-3001) (Washington, DC: National Center for Health Services Research, 1983).

13. J.S. Gonnella et al., "Use of Outcome Measures in Ambulatory Care Evaluation," in: *Ambulatory Medical Care Quality Assurance*, eds. G.A. Giebink and H.H. White (La Jolla, CA: La Jolla Health Science Publications, 1977), pp.91-125.

14. M.L. Garg et al., "Evaluating Inpatient Costs: The Staging Mechanism," *Medical Care*, 16 (1981): 191-201.

15. The development of approaches for use of disease staging to analyze timing of hospitalization was funded by the W.K. Kellogg Foundation, Battle Creek, MI.

16. Garg, "Evaluating Inpatient Costs," pp. 191-201.

17. Gonnella, "The Staging Concept," pp. 13-21.

18. Gonnella, "Use of Outcome Measures," pp. 91-125.

19. P.O. Grimaldi and J.A. Micheletti, *Diagnosis Related Groups: A Practitioner's Guide* (Chicago: Pluribus Press, 1982).

20. J.E. Conklin et al., "Disease Staging: Implications for Hospital Reimbursement and Management," *Health Care Financing Review* Suppl., 1984 (November).

21. Gonnella, "Staging of Disease," pp. 637-644.

22. Gonnella, "The Staging Concept," pp.13-21.

23. Gonnella, "Use of Outcome Measures," pp. 911-125.

24. Grimaldi, *Diagnosis Related Groups*.

25. J. Fothergill, "An Account of the Sore Throat with Ulcers," in: *Classic Studies of Infectious Disease*, ed. L.A. May (Oceanside, NY: Dabor Science Publications, 1977).

26. Ibid.

Chapter 4

The Science of Prediction and Its Implications for Quality Assessment in Intensive Care*

William A. Knaus, M.D.

I would like to begin this chapter by taking us back to the sixteenth century and the small Italian town of Capodistria, located on a small island some fifteen miles from Trieste. It was here in 1561 that an Italian physician, Santorio Santorio, was born. Santorio was a friend and contemporary of Galileo and was educated and practicing medicine at the peak of Italian scientific influence when medical schools such as Pavia and Padua were considered the best in the world.

The medicine that was taught at Padua, however, was not uniquely or even predominantly Italian. Until the 1600s the main source of medical knowledge was Greek--predominantly the works of the ancient Greek physician, Galen. Galen was a brilliant and extraordinarily important figure in medical history.

He helped establish the scientific study of anatomy and he gave medicine the humoral theory of health and disease, the concept that every body contained four elementary humors--hot, cold, dry, and moist--and that the relative balance among these four determined a person's state of health.

Of Galen's many contributions, the humoral theory of disease was the most powerful, influencing medical practice for sixteen centuries. No one seriously challenged this theory until Santorio, through his friendship with Galileo, became aware of attempts to measure changes in the earth's atmosphere using a new device called a thermoscope. Santorio helped adopt these measurement principles to medicine with the development and use of one of the earliest thermometers. By the use of this and similar devices, Santorio demonstrated, for the first time, that patients were not absolutely

---

*Copyright held by the author.

hot or cold, as Galen had claimed, but had distinct and measurable temperatures. This knowledge fundamentally changed the practice of medicine.[1]

As long as medicine was ruled by Galen's theory of the four humors, elements that were absolute and meaningful only for one individual, there could never be any quantitative way of comparing the conditions of one individual with another or against a reference standard. Santorio showed, however, that not only temperature but also heart rate and metabolism, other elements that were thought absolute and unquantifiable, could be measured. Precise measurement formed the basis of physiology and modern medical practice.

Let us now shift to the twentieth century. Think for a moment that American medicine is as advanced in its time as Italian medicine was in the era of Galileo and Santorio. I recently gave a presentation at one of the prominent medical centers in the United States, equivalent in reputation to Padua in the sixteenth century. I was speaking about the science of prediction and how the precise measurement of patient outcomes could create a new era of medical research and policy. One of the comments I received, a fairly typical one, was that prediction in medicine was impossible. I was told that "a patient's prognosis is either black or white; they are going to live or they are going to die."

This kind of bias was precisely what physicians in Santorio's time were saying about the four humors--a patient is either hot *or* cold, moist *or* dry. It wasn't true then and it isn't now. The patients we treat have discrete and measurable temperatures and heart rates. They also have quantifiable predictions of outcome. Like temperature and pulse, these predictions are dynamic; they change as the result of treatment and the patient's response to that treatment.

Being able to measure and record these outcome estimates, both before as well as during the course of therapy, can, as I will discuss, give us insights into the most appropriate use of advanced medical care. Thus, I believe it is time for the medical profession to take up the 2,000-year-old challenge of scientific prediction. As Peter Medawar commented, "A science does not truly become mature until it develops a predictive capability."[2] While I do not expect medicine to develop a predictive capability similar to the exact sciences of physics and chemistry to which Medawar was alluding, I agree with Alvan Feinstein, who recently wrote, "The omission of prediction from the major goals of medical science has impoverished the intellectual content of clinical work since a modern clinician's main challenge in the care of patients is to make predictions."[3]

One might respond that such predictions have always been the foundation of good medical practice. However, I would emphasize that when all the tools and drugs a physician controlled could be placed in his small black leather bag, therapeutic choices were few, and prediction could be left an informal undertaking largely drawn from the physician's personal experience. The scope of modern medical practice is now far beyond the limits of a black bag. It is interventionist, institutional, and intricate. It is driven by a rapidly expanding base of theoretical information and new technologies; its proper practice increasingly requires corporate, rather than individual, leadership; and its complexity is producing questions of allocation of scarce resources to which we do not have good answers. These changes in medical practice cannot be addressed by looking back to romantic models of past behavior.

These changes in medical practice have produced four new challenges that previous generations never had to face. These four changes are the reasons *why* we need to take up the science of prediction. They are:

1). The challenge of precisely measuring the incremental value of technologically advanced medical care.
2). The challenge of convincing ourselves and others that new technologies are really better.
3). The challenge of precisely measuring the quality of our performance on both an institutional and individual level.
4). Improving the precision of our outcome predictions for individual patients--our most difficult challenge of all.

These four challenges can be thought of as four major objectives for prognostic research. I would like to use them as an outline for a discussion of the science of prediction. Before doing that, however, I would like to begin with a few principles of how we might begin that exploration.

The first principle is: what should we be predicting? Because much of modern medical and surgical care concentrates on the treatment of very ill patients--patients with a high risk of dying--health policy increasingly focuses on the release of hospital mortality data. (See Chapters 1, 2 and 7.) We should thus begin our predictive efforts with hospital mortality. This is not to conclude that we should only be concerned with mortality--the quality and length of survival is also important--but let us start our efforts with prediction of hospital mortality.

The second principle is: when should we be performing the predictions? We want our predictions to be available before the end. We need them to be available prior to treatment or, at the very least, shortly after we begin therapy.

We also want any method we choose to be reliable so that when different persons apply it to patients with different diseases, the results are consistent. We need a sensible system that can be applied directly to the majority of acutely ill patients, and we want it to be suitable. In other words, the system should not be dependent on therapy or physician judgments, since we will be using the results of our analysis to judge the quality of these decisions. The latter is a key conceptual point. Finally, we want the method to work well--it must be repeatedly and independently validated to outcome in new groups of patients.

With these principles in mind, let us look at one model of how we might start to predict hospital outcome for severely ill patients. At our current level of understanding, we believe that outcome from an acute illness is determined by four patient factors: the patients' *disease,* their *physiologic reserve,* which encompasses considerations of age and chronic health status, the *acute severity* of their disease, and, finally, their *response to treatment* (Figure 1).

A patient's outcome is also influenced by four treatment factors: 1) the type of treatment available; 2) its organization; 3) its timing; and 4) its process, or the manner in which physicians, nurses, and others work together to apply it. It has been very difficult to determine the value of these different aspects of treatment because we have not fully described our patients. But let us now take this model and see what its implications are for the four key questions we listed at the beginning of this chapter.

The first question is how we can use the science of prognosis to more precisely measure the value of technologically advanced medical care. Our inability to document more fully the incremental value of modern medical care has created confusion in both medicine and public policy. For example, we frequently hear comments and read articles concluding that the probability of a good outcome is inversely related to the amount of medical treatment.[4] "The more treatment, the worse the outcome," and "the mortality rate is directly related to the number of tubes and lines," are remarks that tend to disparage the value of advanced medical care, can lead to overly pessimistic prognoses, and encourage the thinking that a patient must receive a certain type and duration of therapy before a prognosis is established. But recall that an analysis that uses therapy to predict outcome fails to account for any of our important patient risks factors. To illustrate this point, we published a study a few years ago that first plotted the simple relationship between treatment, as measured by the total number of therapeutic intervention scoring system, or TISS, points a group of intensive care unit (ICU) patients received, and their hospital mortality.[5] We found, as others had, that the more treatment a patient received, the worse the outcome. We also had the ability in this data base, however, to estimate each patient's severity of illness at the time he or she initially presented for ICU treatment. When this variable is added to the analysis, we find that we have a much different and much more satisfying outcome (Figure 2 and Figure 3).

The relationship, once controlled for the initial severity of the patient, suggests that there are ICU patients that will die quickly before they have received much treatment, another group of patients whose survival actually decreases with increased treatment, and then, at the extreme range of treatment, a more direct relationship between treatment and survival. We do not claim that this analysis proves that intensive care saves lives, but it does indicate that a more comprehensive model of clinical science produces results which are richer and closer to the actual situation.

Let us now look at some other examples illustrating that prior to treatment predictability of the risk of death of severely ill patients can help us precisely measure the incremental value of treatment. One example comes from the surgical literature on acute burns in an article by Feller and associates.[6] They showed that knowing the patient's age (a key element of their physiologic reserve) and the percent of the body that is severely burned, one can calculate a pretreatment risk of death. By then looking at such estimates over time, one can see that improvements in burn care treatment resulted in improved probabilities of survival for patients with severe life-threatening injuries treated in the late 1970s, compared to the late 1960s.

A second, and even more dramatic, example of improvement over time can be seen in an analysis of neonatal death rates by Philip.[7] The gestational age and the birth weight of a neonate are excellent pretreatment predictors of the risk of death. Philip and his associates demonstrate substantial progress in saving the lives of very low birth weight infants over time, comparing the initial 1958 data from Colorado with 1976 information from Vermont. It was information like this that encouraged the spread of regional neonatal services and resulted in a corresponding nationwide improvement in the quality of care. Think of what the implications would be if we had similar predictive abilities in other disciplines. If we did, we could take advantage of many natural experiments, both over time and between centers, to pinpoint the value of new technology.

Unfortunately, at the same time neonatologists were deservedly patting themselves on the back for the progress they had made, other specialties were struggling. For example, in an article on the initial seven years of experience at the University of Colorado's respiratory ICU[8], data indicated there had been substantial progress in the technical and therapeutic capabilities of advanced respiratory care, certainly ones equivalent to those we have just reviewed in burn and neonatal care. Yet the crude, or unadjusted for severity, mortality rates reported in this article demonstrated no improvement. Was this true, or was there a more appropriate conclusion, the one suggested by the article's authors, that they were treating more severely ill patients in 1974 than in 1968 and doing better? Without a pretreatment prediction, it was impossible to tell.

To address this problem and the overall challenge of prognosis, my colleagues and I began a research effort in 1978 to design a reliable, sensible, and valid classification system that could be applied to the majority of seriously ill patients. The result of our work is APACHE, a severity of disease classification system.[9] APACHE stands for Acute Physiology and Chronic Health Evaluation. It has been revised once and is now called APACHE II.[10] Following closely our predictive model, the APACHE II severity of disease classification system has three components: an Acute Physiology Score (APS), which summarizes the degree of acute physiologic abnormalities to measure the acute severity of disease, along with a chronic health assessment which uses age, and chronic diseases to estimate an individual's physiologic reserve. The sum of the parts is a cardinal index score that varies from zero to seventy-one, with a usual range of zero to fifty. An increasing score is strongly associated with an increasing acute risk of death. The APACHE II scoring system has been validated in thousands of acutely ill patients in many hospitals throughout this country and around the world. In each case, there is a strong and predictable relationship between the initial APACHE II score at the time of ICU admission and subsequent hospital outcome. Thus, the APACHE II score can be thought of as a comprehensive risk stratification or predictive system applicable to adults with a variety of acute life-threatening diseases.

The APACHE II score is meant to be used in combination with a precise description of the patient's disease, because the implications of acute physiologic abnormalities, as measured by the Acute Physiology Score (APS) component of the APACHE II scoring system, are not equivalent in all diseases. For example, patients with septic shock, a disease whose exact pathophysiology is poorly understood, have a higher death rate at any level of physiologic disturbance than patients with drug overdoses, a better understood disease.

We recently published information, however, suggesting that there may be a consistent underlying relationship between acute changes in physiologic balance and the patient's subsequent risk of death.[11] Figure 4 illustrates the relationship between the initial and actual patient outcomes for six common medical diagnoses. These results show that, while the intercept of the line relating changes in initial physiologic balance to outcome varies among diagnoses, the slope of each line (i.e., the incremental increase in death rate for increase in APS) is identical to about a 2 percent rise in death rate for every one point rise in APS. We have now found this same relationship in thirty-four different, acute, life-threatening diseases.

A number of investigators are beginning to use this predictive capability to better determine the efficacy of new therapies or new combinations of existing treatments. The APS is being used extensively by gastrointestinal surgeons, for example, to evaluate the efficacy of various antibiotic regimens or percutaneous versus surgical drainage for treatment of intra-abdominal abscesses.[12]

The area where this research has had its greatest visibility, however, is in its ability to uncover important variations in the quality of care--especially intensive care--among different hospitals. A particularly relevant study was one in which my colleagues and I evaluated outcome from intensive care in major medical center hospitals.[13] It contained information on 5,030 ICU admissions from thirteen major U.S. medical centers and their nineteen ICUs. Some are very well-known academic medical centers; others are large nonteaching hospitals. All volunteered to take part in this study.

At each of the centers, we studied a random sample of patients. For each patient, we collected information on diagnosis, surgical status, the patient's physiologic reserve, and severity of disease using our APACHE II classification system. APACHE II scoring was done at the time of the patient's ICU admission, prior to substantial treatment. We also followed all patients for their response to treatment and for their outcome in terms of mortality at hospital discharge.

To evaluate other factors impacting on patient outcome, we collected information from each center on their technical capability in terms of therapy available and their organizational structure, (i.e., how the unit was run). To monitor the timing and nature of treatment decisions, we followed each patient each day for the type and amount of therapy provided in the form of daily TISS recordings. We then used the patient risk factors of diagnosis, surgical status, and APACHE II score to stratify patients at ICU admission by their estimated risk of death using the experience of the entire group as the standard. In other words, we used the group experience to provide for each patient an estimated risk of death based upon the outcome of other patients with similar characteristics.

The results of that analysis are shown in Figure 5, where we have ranked the 5,030 patients by their relative risk of hospital death. For each three-point increase in APACHE II score, there is a significant increase in the predicted probability of hospital death. This predicted risk closely matches the observed death rates. This finding is consistent throughout the range of mortality from low to middle to high. The correlation between groups of observed and predicted death rates is very high, with an overall correlation coefficient of .995.

Next we used this predictive ability to estimate group death rates for each of the thirteen hospitals and then compared each institution's actual versus predicted mortality rates. The results are given in Table 1. In the first column, the hospitals are listed from one to thirteen. The crude hospital death rate appears in the third column. This column illustrates that mortality rates unadjusted for patient severity are not helpful in judging outcome. The figures in this column have no relation to a hospital's performance. In subsequent columns, there are two examples of each hospital's mortality ratio--first for nonoperative patients and then for all patients.

The mortality ratio is the ratio of observed or actual deaths over the number predicted using each patient's APACHE II score, surgical status, and disease. Hospitals with a ratio of one are performing at the average for the sample, (i.e., their observed and predicted deaths match closely). Those with a ratio less than one are performing better than average; those with ratios greater than one are performing below average. After controlling for all major patient risk factors, one hospital does significantly better than all others (Hospital 1), and one (Hospital 13) does significantly worse. These variations are found in both medical patients and total patients. They are not solely the result of variations in surgical skills.

Remember that, for each of these hospitals, the predicted death rates were obtained using the experience of the entire group as the reference; thus, these hospitals are being directly compared to each other. Although all thirteen hospitals volunteered for comparison, we found their performance in the quality of care was not the same.

We found that the amount and type of therapy, as well as the formal organization of the unit, did not correlate with each hospital's relative performance when we explored variations in these thirteen hospitals. The type of therapy did not correlate, because all of the units did not use common ICU therapies such as ventilators, vasoactive drugs, and pulmonary artery catheters with equal frequency. Each hospital's formal organizational structure also did not relate with performance. It is true that Hospital 1 was a teaching hospital with a full-time ICU director, and Hospital 13 was a nonteaching hospital with part-time leadership. But Hospitals 2 and 3 were also nonteaching institutions, and Hospital 12 was a large teaching hospital. Therefore, what we inferred was that the hospital that performed better than all others in this study had the best system for coordination between physician and nursing staffs. The hospital with the poorest performance lacked all elements of a good interaction among staff. We reached this conclusion because the variation we found in the degree of staff coordination was the greatest single difference between the best- and worst-performing institutions.

For example, the ICU of Hospital 1 used carefully designed clinical protocols implemented by senior level in-unit physicians who had major responsibility for all patient care. The highly trained and educated nursing staff of Hospital 1 was given independent responsibilities within the protocols. This independent authority included the right to cancel major elective surgery if adequate ICU resources did not exist to treat the patient after the operation.

At the other exteme was the ICU at Hospital 13 which, during the time of this study, had very poor communication between physician and nursing staff, with disagreements over the appropriateness of assigned work loads, difficulty with the ongoing care of patients requiring long-term ventilation, and frequent complications from invasive procedures. In contrast to Hospital 1, the physicians and nurses in Hospital 13 also wouldn't sit in the same room together.

Since this was our initial effort at multi-institutional comparison, however, we emphasize that our conclusions concerning exactly what prompted the differences in mortality performance are tentative. Other causal possibilities include the quality of the medical staff or the type of leadership. Each of these factors needs to be examined in a larger random national study, one that is now in its final design phase.

This new effort will also provide us with representative national performance-level mortality data to which all our nation's ICUs can be compared. We will be able to do this because we can prognostically stratify patients at ICU admission by their estimated risk of death.

How much variation in quality might we find? The evidence from our thirteen hospital study, as well as two other recent surveys, suggests that it may be substantial. In the first of these reports, Dr. Mary Ellen Avery of Harvard and colleagues compared the incident of chronic obstructive lung disease (COLD) among survivors of neonatal care at eight university medical centers.[14] The proportion of low birth-weight neonates who survive but have serious lung problems is a very precise and important outcome measure of the quality of care. They found that, among the eight centers, there was one that had statistically fewer survivors with COLD than the other seven centers. The reason? It is not certain, but the best performing center was the only one that had a single physician in charge of all respiratory care given these neonates.

The second, and more disturbing, report is one produced recently by the federal Centers for Disease Control.[15] While investigating the care given by an ICU nurse in Prince George's County, MD, who was accused of murdering four patients, the CDC found that, over a fifteen-month period, the nurse in question had fifty-six cardiac arrests occur under her supervision. By comparison, fourteen of her nursing colleagues who worked similar shifts and an equivalent number of hours had no more than four. Most had only one or two patients who suffered a cardiac arrest.

The need for explicit outcome criteria is also supported by recent findings suggesting that relying on the personal observations of hospital administrators and physicians to monitor quality and make adjustments may not always result in the best decisions. We are beginning to understand that the important choices and decisions most individuals (including physicians) make are really not decisions arrived at after analytically weighing alternatives, but are habits encouraged by widely accepted but seldom examined group values. Such a decision-making process forecloses many alternatives because of our comparison of probabilities--something that is beyond everyday human capabilities.

This observation leads us to another goal for the science of prediction--namely, improving outcome predictions for individual patients. To be able to accurately predict outcomes for individuals, we must first acknowledge that the factors determining outcomes for groups of patients and for individual patients are identical. However, when we speak about individuals, the precision of our predictions must be great, and the confidence we have in these estimates must be high. At the current level of understanding, prognostic estimates based on information available prior to treatment enables us to confidently identify specific outcome situations in only a small number of patients. We are frequently still obligated to treat many patients in order to determine their response to therapy.

A study from Saudi Arabia relates to this issue. The study, recently published in *Lancet,* used changes in the acute physiology score over time to identify patients whose initial response to intensive treatment suggested that additional treatment with another scarce resource--in this case, total parenteral nutrition--might not be helpful.[16]

We believe that such studies, when combined with other patient risk factors and good clinical judgment, could potentially improve the quality of our decision making. For one thing, it could help us avoid what Professor Jennett has called the vicious cycle of commitment when future therapy is initiated, not because of its expected value, but only because past therapy has failed.[17] It could also help us ensure that future medical allocation and rationing decisions are based on the ability of patients to benefit, rather than ability to pay. However, before such studies can be used at the bedside, much more basic research work needs to be done.

In conclusion, what are the implications of this type of research on clinical prediction for American medicine? First, I think we should realize that just as the measurements of temperature and pulse proposed by Santorio did not become commonplace for over a century, many of the goals I set forward at the beginning of this chapter will require much more work before they can become part of the mainstream of medical practice.

However, there are some immediate objectives that we can aim for and reach now. There are now important variations in our ability to treat the sick, and anticipating that our future progress will bring even more complexity to medical care, it is likely that institutional variations in quality will become more common and more important. Therefore, the challenge for us is to identify quality in a way that is fair and accurate. One way is to develop a national mortality-based outcome standard for all adult medical-surgical ICUs. By collecting data from a representative sample of U.S. hospitals and their intensive care units, we can provide realistic expectations of performance and new insights to ensure that there are more hospitals at the high level of Hospital 1 and fewer performing like Hospital 13. If we are right in our estimates of the variation in quality among various ICUs, such a national effort could potentially save the lives of thousands of critically ill patients each year.

Figure 1. Determinants of outcome from an acute illness.

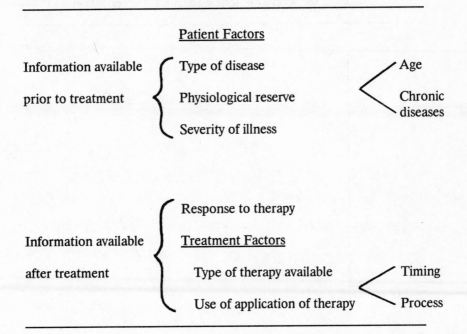

Figure 2. Relationship between treatment and survival. Not controlling for severity of illness (derived from equation #1).

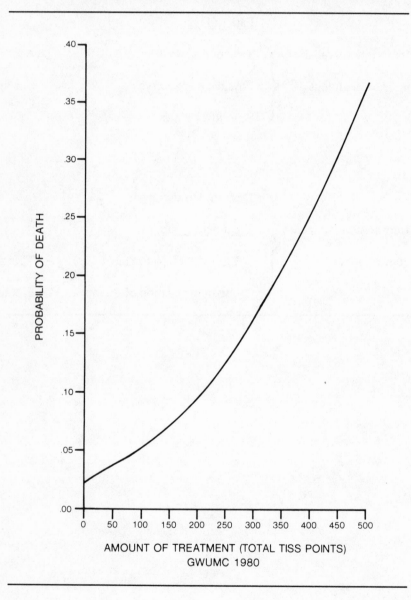

Figure 3. Relationship between treatment and survival with and without control for severity of illness.

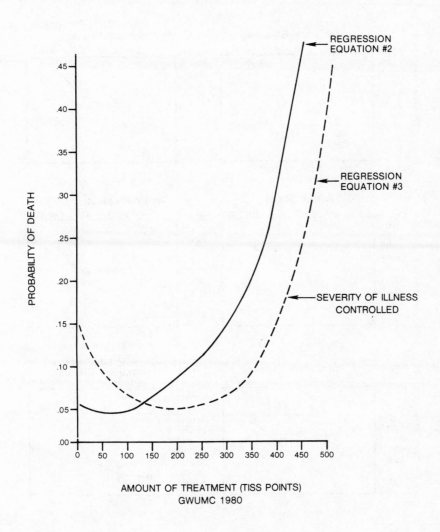

PROBABILITY OF DEATH

REGRESSION
EQUATION #2

REGRESSION
EQUATION #3

SEVERITY OF ILLNESS
CONTROLLED

AMOUNT OF TREATMENT (TISS POINTS)
GWUMC 1980

Figure 4. Relationship between increasing severity of disease (Acute Physiology Score [APS]-12) and hospital death rate for six acute diseases.

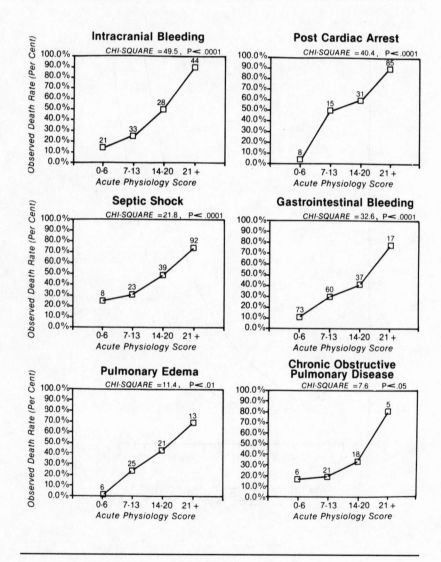

Figure 5. Apache II scores and observed death rates.

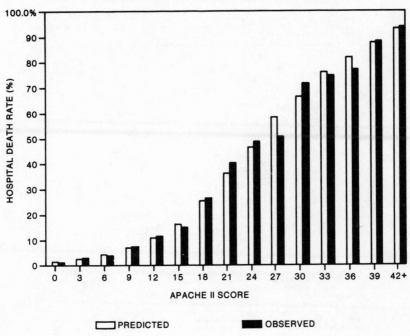

Table 1

Comparison of Observed and Predicted Hospital Deaths: 5,030 Intensive Care Unit Admissions to 13 Hospitals

Hospital performance ranking	Total number admissions	Hospital death rate (percent)	Non-Operative Admissions			All Admissions		
			Number observed deaths	Number predicted deaths	Mortality ratio	Number observed deaths	Number predicted deaths	Mortality ratio
1	365	11.2	30 /	46 =	0.65[*]	41 /	69 =	0.59[*]
2+	201	20.4	32 /	34 =	0.93	41 /	49 =	0.84
3+	159	18.9	20 /	23 =	0.87	30 /	34 =	0.88
4	201	38.3	77 /	86 =	0.90	77 /	86 =	0.90++
5	500	9.8	20 /	17 =	1.18	49 /	53 =	0.92
6	426.	8.9	21 /	21 =	1.00	38 /	41 =	0.93
7	412	17.2	54 /	58 =	0.93	71 /	74 =	0.96
8	198	19.7	33 /	37 =	0.94	39 /	39 =	1.00
9	1,657	24.1	269 /	263 =	1.02	400 /	383 =	1.04
10	366	14.8	20 /	15 =	1.33	54 /	49 =	1.10
11	170	26.5	39 /	34 =	1.14	45 /	40 =	1.13
12	178	31.5	44 /	37 =	1.18	56 /	44 =	1.27
13+	197	26.4	38 /	21 =	1.81[*]	52 /	33 =	1.58[*]

[*] $p < .01$. Computed as a t-test of the difference between two means. (An alternate analysis including institutional effects in the estimated logistic regression equation yielded similar institutional differences and larger significance levels for each institution; e.g., Chi-square = 24.6, p < .0001 for Hospital 1 and Chi-square = 15.4, p < .0001 for Hospital 13.)

+ Nonteaching hospitals.

++ p = .03, Chi-square = 4.6 in the multivariate logistic regression equation.

Predicted deaths were computed as the sum of individual risks with a multiple logistic regression equation. Non-operative predicted deaths were computed from a separate analysis of those patients.

NOTES

1.   R.H. Major, "Santorio Santorio," *Annals of Medical History*, 101 (1938):369-381.

2.   P. Medawar, *The Limits of Science* (Cambridge: Oxford University Press, 1984).

3.   A.R. Feinstein, "An Additional Basic Science for Clinical Medicine: The Constraining Fundamental Paradigms," *Annals of Internal Medicine*, 99 (1983):393.

4.   J.M. Civetta, "The Inverse Relationship Between Cost and Survival," *Journal of Surgical Residency*, 14 (1973): 265-269.

5.   R. A. Schefler et al., "Severity of Illness and the Relationship Between Intensive Care and Survival," *American Journal of Public Health*, 72 (1982):449-454.

6.   I. Feller, D. Tholen, and R.G. Cornell, "Improvements in Burn Care 1965-1979, *Journal of the American Medical Association*, 244 (1980):2074-2078.

7.   A.G.S. Philip et al., "Neonatal Mortality Risk for the Eighties: The Importance of Birth Weight/Gestational Age Groups," *Pediatrics*, 58(1981):122.

8.   T.L. Petty et al., "Intensive Respiratory Care Unit: Review of Ten Years Experience," *Journal of the American Medical Association*, 34(1975):233.

9.   W.A. Knaus et al., "APACHE -- Acute Physiology and Chronic Health Evaluation: A Physiologically Based Classification System," *Critical Care Medicine*, 9(1981):591-597.

10. W.A. Knaus et al., "APACHE II: A Severity of Disease Classification System," *Critical Care Medicine*, 13(1985): 818-829.

11.   D.P. Wagner, W.A. Knaus, and E. A. Draper, "Physiologic Abnormalities and Outcome from Acute Disease," *Archives of Internal Medicine*, 146 (1986): 1389-1396.

12.   E.P. Dellinger et al., "Surgical Infection Stratification System for Intra-Abdominal Infection Multicenter Trial," *Archives of Surgery*, 120 (1985):21-29.

13.   W.A. Knaus et al., "An Evaluation of Outcome from Intensive Care in Major Medical Centers," *Annals of Internal Medicine*, 104(1986):410-418.

14.   M.E. Avery, W.H. Tooley, and J.B. Keeler, "Is Chronic Disease in Low Birth Weight Infants Preventable? A Survey of Eight Centers," *Pediatrics* ,79 (1987):26-30.

15.   J. Sacks, *Cluster of Unexplained Deaths at a Hospital in Maryland* (CDC Report no. SPI-17).

16.   R.W.S Chang, S. Jacobs, and B. Lee, "Use of APACHE II Severity of Disease Classification to Identify Intensive Care Patients Who Would Not Benefit from Total Parenteral Nutrition," *Lancet*, II (1986):1483-1486.

17.   B. Jennett, "Inappropriate Use of Intensive Care," *British Medical Journal*, 289(1984):1709-1711.

Chapter 5

History and Mission of Quality Assurance in the Public Sector

Andrew Webber

The public sector's participation in the medical care system has been characterized by two distinct emphases: broadening access to medical care services and, more recently, containing medical care costs. This chapter explores what I hope will become the next major theme in national health policy: assuring the quality of medical care. Several factors are pushing the quality issue to the forefront at this time:

1). The present emphasis on cost containment heightens public concern regarding potential compromises to quality of care. Reimbursement reforms, such as the Medicare Prospective Payment System (PPS) and the spread of prepaid health plans invite concerns about underservice and selective enrollment;

2). In an increasingly competitive medical marketplace, quality becomes a distinguishing feature among competitors. Providers strive to deliver high-quality services while consumers, facing choices in the marketplace, search for information on provider quality; and

3). Medical practice variation, reflecting uncertainty in medical decision making and the need to build a knowledgeable consensus among practitioners regarding the appropriateness of various therapies, suggests opportunities for service reduction with accompanying improvements in quality.

Elevating quality assurance to prominence in the national policy debate will not be easy. Quality is an elusive concept in medical care, meaning very different things to different people. (See Chapters

1 and 14.) Two primary challenges emerge: the development of objective and scientifically valid tools to measure quality (quality assessment); and the implementation of educational and, when necessary, punitive interventions to motivate positive changes in practice behavior (quality assurance). (See Chapters 2, 6 and 8.) To meet these challenges will require innovation, the commitment of resources, and political will.

This chapter outlines the past, present, and future role of the public sector in quality assurance activities. The Peer Review Organization (PRO) program is the centerpiece of the federal government's efforts to assure quality medical care in its Medicare and Medicaid programs, and it will be highlighted in this discussion.

HISTORY

Over the last 50 years, the public sector's efforts with respect to quality medical care have focused on broadening access to it. Though easily forgotten in this present era of cost containment, the thrust of the federal government's health policy, beginning with World War II and extending into the 1960s, was to encourage expansion of the medical care industry. To accomplish this goal, policies and programs were implemented, including the following:

1). the tax deductibility of employer-sponsored health insurance coverage. The favorable tax treatment of insurance coverage encouraged the spread and comprehensiveness of health benefits in the private sector;

2). the Hill-Burton program which established strong incentives for hospital development even in the remotest of communities;

3). the Medicare and Medicaid programs to provide access to basic medical care services for the elderly and the indigent; and

4). direct and indirect subsidies for medical education, dramatically increasing the supply of physicians and other health care professionals.

These federal initiatives were highly successful in realizing their goal of broadening access to care. Unfortunately, they fueled an explosive growth in the medical care industry and led, predictably, to spiraling health care costs. Starting in the 1970s, a weakened American economy and the stark reality of growing federal deficits combined to end the government's expansionist role. No longer were new benefits or provider subsidies economically and politically feasible.

In contrast to these efforts to expand access, the public sector's role in assuring the quality of medical care has, until recent times, been largely governed by a policy of laissez-faire. Until the establishment of the Medicare and Medicaid programs in the 1960's, public entities uniformly deferred to the medical profession in matters regarding quality assurance. The only significant traditional involvement of the public sector in quality assurance entailed the system of medical licensure. Enabling legislation at the state level conferred authority upon a state board of medical examiners to license physicians. State licensing boards were also empowered to suspend and revoke licenses based on evidence of unethical practice and the provision of poor-quality care.

MEDICARE AND MEDICAID

In 1965, Congress enacted the Medicare and Medicaid legislation to broaden access to care for the poor and elderly. Congress signaled its concern for assuring the quality of care in these programs principally through two important program features: the conditions of participation and the survey and certification program.

Conditions of Participation

Under law, providers are required as a condition of participation in the Medicare and Medicaid programs to comply with certain obligations. The program requires that reimbursed services be: provided economically and only when, and to the extent, they are medically necessary; and of a quality that meets professionally recognized standards of health care.

In addition to these general provisions, there are many specific conditions of participation in the Medicare/Medicaid programs that relate to quality. For instance, many of the standards for hospital accreditation established by the Joint Commission on Accreditation of Healthcare Organizations (JCAHO) became incorporated into the conditions of participation. Examples include physical plant safety requirements, the establishment of hospital quality assurance committees, and guidelines for the structure and responsibilities of hospital medical staffs. Over the years, various conditions of participation have been added to the Medicare/Medicaid programs. As late as the Omnibus Budget Reconciliation Act of 1986, requirements for a hospital discharge planning process were established as a condition of participation. The impetus for this provision grew directly from public concerns about the impact of the incentives in Medicare's PPS on hospital discharge policies.

Survey and Certification

The first initiative the federal government established to monitor actual compliance with Medicare/Medicaid conditions of participation was the survey and certification program. Modeled after the JCAHO survey system, its purpose was to assure that hospitals and nursing homes participating in Medicare were conducive environments for the provision of quality services. Survey teams were discharged to hospitals to conduct onsite inspections and used the conditions of participation as the basis for measuring program compliance.

The conditions of participation and the survey and certification program provided a needed first step in the federal government's direct involvement in assuring quality of care. Neither effort, however, could assure that medical care services were, in fact, delivered appropriately and with good quality. At best, the survey process measured whether a hospital, by virtue of its internal organization and structure, was capable of delivering quality services. It could not measure whether the process and outcomes of patient care were acceptable.

PROFESSIONAL STANDARD REVIEW ORGANIZATIONS

By 1972, seven years after the enactment of the Medicare legislation, it had become clear to Congress that the costs of the program were far surpassing original assumptions. Senate Finance Committee hearings uncovered widespread evidence that medical claims were being processed by fiscal intermediaries in which the services were either never provided or were medically unnecessary. Congress, led by the efforts of Senator Wallace Bennett (R-UT), became convinced that a more thorough examination of the actual provision of services was needed. It was also apparent to lawmakers that the physician community and not fiscal intermediaries needed to participate in the medical review of services. Senator Bennett argued that only physicians were in a position to pass judgment on the appropriateness and quality of medical care services. In 1972, P.L. 92-603 was enacted, establishing the Professional Standards Review Organization (PSRO) program. The program's stated purpose was to assure that the two primary obligations of the provider community participating in Medicare were being met: 1) that services were being provided economically and only when medically necessary; and, 2) that services were of a quality that met professionally recognized standards of health care.

The PSRO program had several important features:

- By design, PSROs were nonprofit, physician run, and locally based organizations. Nationwide, over 200 PSROs were established within the program. In larger states like California, over 20 different review areas were established.

- PSROs were funded by yearly grants through the Congressional appropriations process.

- The criteria and standards established by PSROs were locally based.

- The focus of review efforts was on hospital based services, particularly length of stay and use of ancillary services. PSROs experimented with review of ambulatory services and nursing homes, but this activity was never widely incorporated into the program.

- The conduct of Medical Care Evaluation (MCE) studies formed the nucleus for review of quality of care. (See Chapters 2 and 6.)

- Much of PSRO review was "delegated" to the hospital. Hospital review committees actually conducted the review of services, with the review organizations monitoring the effectiveness of these committees. Many argued that this delegation placed hospitals in an untenable conflict of interest and represented a major weakness of the program.

■ PSRO review of services was conducted on an exhaustive case-by-case basis through review of medical records. First-level reviewers applied clinical criteria, and cases not meeting the criteria were referred to a physician for a final determination. Only a physician could decide that a medical service was unnecessary or did not meet professionally recognized standards of quality.

■ A comprehensive clinical abstract data system was created to permit PSROs to aggregate medical record information and profile practice behavior. This led, in time, to the opportunity to "focus" or "target" review rather than review all cases or a random sample of cases.

■ PSROs were allowed only to recommend denials of payment to the fiscal intermediary and could not make the final determination to do so. The hospital community was also successful in petitioning for a "waiver of liability" provision under the PSRO program. In seeking this waiver, hospitals argued that only physicians were in a position to judge the appropriateness of services so hospitals should not be held liable for adverse review decisions until certain percentages or thresholds of denied care had been reached. This "favorable presumption" that hospitals could not have known that services delivered in their own facility were unnecessary translated into few payment denials during the PSRO program.

■ PSROs were given the authority to recommend to the federal government the exclusion of practitioners and providers from the Medicare program based on grossly inadequate provision of care.

The PSRO program, so designed, faced a stormy decade. From the very beginning of the program, organized medicine feared that PSRO was a disguise for government efforts to control costs rather than improve quality. Political acceptance by the medical community thus virtually evaporated as the government's cost containment agenda became increasingly apparent. Evaluations of the PSRO program conducted by the Congressional Budget Office concluded that program costs were as great as the savings realized by review activities. This finding was not surprising given the design of the program. By the late 1970s and early 1980s, the Congressional Appropriation Committees had grown increasingly skeptical of PSRO program effectiveness. The only vocal support for the PSRO program came from large corporations, represented by the Washington Business Group on Health, who testified in Congressional hearings that review contracts with local PSROs had been a successful component of their cost management strategies. Significantly, the beneficiary community was not a vocal supporter. The quality issue had not reached the critical importance it would with the introduction of prospective payment. (See Chapter 7.)

Ronald Reagan's election to office in 1980 added to the chorus of PSRO criticism. President Reagan's first budget called for the phase out of the PSRO program along with the health planning program. The Administration cited four reasons for its opposition to PSRO:

1). The program was regulatory, and the Administration wanted to introduce greater competition to the medical care industry;

2). The program had not been cost effective;

3). Federal deficits argued for policies to eliminate unnecessary federal spending; and

4). The PSRO medical review function, in the near term, could be better handled by fiscal intermediaries. In this way, a single administrative entity could integrate payment decisions and medical review functions.

Organized medicine applauded this effort to eliminate the PSRO program. The Senate Finance Committee, however, led by the efforts of David Durenberger (R-MN) and Max Baucus (D-MT), was not convinced. Together, they set out to build a new medical review program that responded to the legitimate criticisms of the PSRO program but retained its positive features, including the active participation of the physician community. A full decade after the passage of PSRO, the Durenberger-Baucus effort led to the establishment of the Peer Review Organization (PRO) Program which was enacted into law as a provision of the Tax Equity and Fiscal Responsibility Act of 1982 (TEFRA).

THE PEER REVIEW ORGANIZATION (PRO) PROGRAM

The purpose of the PRO program, like PSRO before it, is to monitor Medicare services to assure that the care delivered is medically necessary and meets professionally recognized standards of quality care. Here, similarities stop. There are six major features of the PRO program that set it apart from earlier PSRO review efforts:

1). Performance-based contracts. There was much criticism of the PSRO program because it was not result-oriented. The federal government never identified its expectations of the review organizations, making evaluation of PSRO efforts difficult, if not impossible. The government was very prescriptive about *how* review should be performed but not *what* it should accomplish. In contrast, the PRO statute makes clear that the federal government would enter "performance based contracts" with PROs driven by a set of negotiated utilization and quality objectives. In return, the government would be less prescriptive about the review process, leaving greater discretion to the PRO to decide how review would be performed.

2). Competitive bidding. Many observers of the PSRO program believed that it "enfranchised" review groups through a system of yearly renewals of federal grants. It was difficult to terminate poor performers, and there was no latitude to reward the best PSROs with expanded responsibilities.

In response to this criticism, the PRO law established a competitive bidding system based on two-year federal contract cycles. The law allowed the federal government to automatically renew contracts with good performers, and, alternatively, seek competitively bid contracts where PRO performance standards were not being met. Both for-profit and not-for-profit organizations would be allowed to compete.

3). Advantage to physician organizations. While not mandating that review must be performed by physician review organizations, the PRO law extended a distinct advantage to physician-based organizations. Fiscal intermediaries were excluded from bidding in the first round of contracts. Thereafter, the Health Care Financing Administration (HCFA), which is responsible for managing the program, must first show that there are no technically acceptable bids from physician organizations before signing a review contract with a fiscal intermediary. At present, there is only one state (Hawaii) where PRO review is being performed by a fiscal intermediary.

4). Consolidation of review areas. Medicaid officials were the first to raise concerns regarding multiple review organizations within one state. Different review philosophies and different standards and criteria employed within a state created administrative nightmares for state-run Medicaid programs. Recognizing this limitation of the PSRO program, the PRO legislation mandated the consolidation of existing review areas. In the regulations for the PRO program, each state was designated as a distinct review area. This consolidation had important implications for the efficiency and consistency of the review process.

5). Nondelegation of review. A major criticism of the PSRO program was the delegation of review to hospitals. The PRO statute remained neutral on this issue, but PRO regulations did not. Arguing that delegation placed hospitals in a conflict of interest, the PRO regulations did not permit delegated review except for quality. In reality, there is presently no delegation of review to hospitals in the PRO program. Thus, with the PRO program, external medical review, independent of the provider or practitioner being reviewed, was implemented for the first time in a federally sponsored review effort.

6). <u>Denial authority and elimination of favorable presumption</u>. Nothing hurt the credibility of PSRO review more than the inability to translate review decisions into meaningful authority. The fact that PRSOs could only recommend payment denials to fiscal intermediaries and the "favorable presumption rule" for hospitals symbolized the program's failings. In response, the PRO statute gave PROs authority to make final payment denial decisions. Regulations released by the Department of Health and Human Services (DHHS) eliminated the favorable presumption rule. Each individual case denial determination now translates into a reduction in payment to hospitals.

The PRO law also tightened the PRO sanction provisions. The law states that a PRO sanction recommendation will stand if the Office of the Inspector General does not make a final determination within 120 days of the recommendation's submission. PSRO sanction recommendations were never acted upon promptly. Taken together, these six provisions grant substantial authority to the PRO program and restore needed credibility to physician peer review efforts.

A year after enactment of the PRO legislation, the Social Security Amendments of 1983 ushered in the Medicare prospective payment system (PPS). Given the implications of this dramatic shift in reimbursement for the incentives facing hospitals, Congress wanted to make certain that PROs would actively oversee the program's implementation and its impact on medical practice. Thus, in the PPS legislation, Congress outlined four specific functions that PROs must perform relative to the new system:

1). <u>Admission review</u>. Because the DRG payment system is based on a fixed price per admission, congressional law makers were concerned that PPS created incentives to increase hospital admissions. If the volume of admissions escalated, cost savings would be jeopardized. Therefore,

Congress mandated that PROs examine the appropriateness and necessity of hospital admissions under PPS. Review of the appropriateness of hospital admission rates was important for another reason. Research data suggested that variations in hospital admission rates were the strongest utilization factor explaining per-capita medical care expenditures. The PSRO program had been criticized for not focusing review efforts on the appropriateness of admissions.

The incentives to reduce hospital length of stay in the new payment system also made clear that PRO review of length of stay and ancillary services would now be unnecessary and none was required. These incentives were, in fact, so strong that within two years of the introduction of PPS there was a two-day reduction in the average length of hospital stay for Medicare beneficiaries. Put another way, hospitals accomplished in that period of time what PSRO's had tried to accomplish over a decade's period.

2).   Quality review.   No longer just rhetoric to appease a nervous medical community, the quality issue moved to center stage as a result of PPS. Given the incentives in PPS, Congress was now legitimately concerned about the potential for underservice. Soon after implementation of PPS, the Senate Aging Committee, chaired by Senator John Heinz (R-PA), held hearings on PPS and quality care. Family members of Medicare beneficiaries testified that their loved ones had been prematurely discharged from hospitals. The quality issue had become an important policy question, galvanizing the interests of the Medicare beneficiary community. (See Chapter 7.) Quality concerns under PPS cemented the political support for an active external quality monitoring system. Such support had not been evident during earlier review efforts. The emergence of this support suggests that, given the increasing stridency of our cost-containment environment, medical review should enjoy long-term political support over time.

The visibility of the quality issue led HCFA to mandate, in the second round of PRO contracts (1986), that PROs apply a generic quality screen to every case under review. (See Chapters 2 and 6). An important element of these screens was the examination of a patient's medical stability at the time of discharge. Though a costly and, in many ways, a blunt instrument, the mandating of quality screens symbolized the emerging importance of the quality issue. For the first time, a balance had been achieved between cost containment and quality assurance goals in the federal government's monitoring of medical care services.

3). Outlier review. PPS created a category of cases called "outliers," in essence representing complex cases for which the standard DRG payment was insufficient. Though a small minority of cases, Congress was concerned with possible manipulation in the designation of outliers and mandated PRO review of them.

4). DRG coding. Similarly, Congress was concerned with hospital manipulation of diagnostic and procedural coding to maximize reimbursement. Such coding forms the basis for the DRG assignment. Obviously, some DRGs have higher weights than others generating greater income to the institution. Therefore, Congress mandated PRO review to assure that the codes assigned to cases match the clinical documentation in the medical record. Whenever a PRO is reviewing a medical record for any reason, e.g., the appropriateness of admission or the quality of care, the medical coding must also be reviewed.

Taken together, these four functions form the nucleus of PRO review activities.

RESULTS OF PRO REVIEW

Evaluating the results of any medical review effort is a complex task. The PRO program is in its infancy, and it will be years before it can be stated confidently whether its efforts are a success or a failure.

The most difficult area of PRO review to assess is the "sentinel" impact of review. How much is practice behavior altered simply because of the presence of PRO review? For example, a sentinel effect may derive from the fact that, on the basis of their review, PROs may deny hospital payments for cases judged to have been inappropriately admitted even after costs have been incurred by an institution. Faced with such external oversight, hospitals have strong incentives to establish their own internal preadmission review systems to assure that only medically necessary and appropriate cases are admitted. It is no surprise then that hospitals have moved ahead with their own utilization review measures. How is the impact of this sentinel effect to be quantified? Similarly, the PRO preadmission certification program will cause physicians to carefully consider their admitting decisions and therein defer some, knowing that they must pass a PRO review. Until such sentinel effects of PRO review are acknowledged and credited to the program, the overall effectiveness of PRO efforts will not be appropriately assessed.

Another troubling evaluation issue is narrow reliance on easily quantified results as the measure of PRO performance. Volume of payment denials and sanctions should not form the basis of evaluation. In fact it contradicts the philosophy of the PRO program. PROs seek improvements in practice behavior through education and peer pressure rather than punitive action. For example, the physician who retires from practice under the pressure of PRO scrutiny or the physician who improves his/her clinical skills by enrolling in a mini-residency program under the supervision of the PRO, represents the real success story of the PRO program. Such outcomes are never recorded in sanction counts, however. Denial and sanction authority is important to establish the authority of the PRO but is used reluctantly when other measures can bring about positive improvements in practice behavior. (See Chapter 6.)

A final reason why the evaluation of PRO review is problematic entails the absence of any meaningful data from the federal government on the results of PRO review. Three years into the program, and even after an entire cycle of PRO contracts has been completed, the federal government has not released to the public any information on PRO impact. What is even more puzzling is that the government requires exhaustive data reports from PROs for every required review activity.

117

Fortunately, the public has access to information on PROs directly from the PRO community. The American Medical Peer Review Association (AMPRA), the national trade association for PROs, has been a consistent source of information on PRO activities and observations. Information gleaned from public testimony by AMPRA officials before Congressional committees and from AMPRA membership surveys can be used to draw some general conclusions about the quality of care under PPS and the state of PRO review:

1). There does not appear to be any widespread evidence that quality has been negatively impacted by the incentives of PPS. In an AMPRA survey, the PRO community was all but unanimous in stating that quality of care has not declined. Some PROs insist that quality of care has improved as hospitals achieve greater efficiencies in internal utilization management.

2). PROs have not found a widespread problem with premature discharges from hospitals. There are reported incidences of premature discharges from hospitals, but they are infrequent and isolated.

3). PROs have uncovered a small percentage of cases that do not meet professionally recognized standards of care. The quality concerns identified in these cases cannot be traced to the new incentives in PPS, but rather are characterized by generalized problems with clinical mismanagement. To date, 104 cases have been forwarded by PROs to the Office of Inspector General (OIG) for sanction. Decisions have been rendered in 62 of these cases; there have been 40 exclusions from the Medicare program and 22 civil monetary penalties have been assessed. The remaining cases are pending final determinations by the OIG or have been returned to the PRO for further investigation.

4). AMPRA has testified that "the major quality of care concern for the Medicare program at this time is the absence of an effective post-acute care and long term care benefit for beneficiaries. At a time when PPS has intensified demand for nonacute care services, benefits have been curtailed." The problem is not that patients are being discharged prematurely, but that medical and support services are not readily available to the discharged patients.

5). Medicare admissions to hospitals have continued to drop, even after experts predicted that admissions would skyrocket under the incentives of PPS. How much PROs have contributed to falling admission rates is debatable. Most experts agree, however, that PRO review has been a factor in the decline. HCFA reports that the national average for PRO denial rates is in the 2 percent to 3 percent range of cases reviewed. (Significantly, even these low rates translate into savings for the Medicare program that exceed PRO program costs.) A continuing question is whether the reduction in inpatient services is causing a corresponding increase in the demand for ambulatory services. Medicare Part B claims have increased since the advent of PPS. For this reason, many believe that a weakness of the PRO program is that its review is confined to the inpatient setting. Early in the program, AMPRA testified that "fiscal constraints on inpatient services created by PPS will encourage the unbundling of hospital services. AMPRA recommends that PROs be given responsibility to review services for Medicare in the ambulatory setting." In response to this concern, Congress passed legislation that will expand PRO review to include: ambulatory surgery, nursing home facilities, home health agencies, and HMOs/CMPs with Medicare risk contracts.

6). PROs have not found review of statistical outliers to be fruitful in terms of uncovering medically unnecessary services. PROs have reported, however, that outlier cases are fertile ground for the identification of quality concerns. Examples have been found of cases with complications that occurred as a result of clinical intervention and not because the case was complex to begin with. This finding raises the importance, in any quality monitoring effort, of classifying patients by the severity of their illness at the point of entry into the medical care system. (See

119

Chapters 2 and 3.) The relationship of medical treatment to clinical outcomes can only be validly evaluated when one knows how sick a patient was to begin with. Similarly, data on the functional status of Medicare beneficiaries is needed upon their entry into nursing homes and other post-acute care settings so that the deterioration or improvement of their functional status over time, a potential indicator of poor or good quality of care in these settings, can be measured.

7).   PROs have not reported widespread evidence of the manipulation of DRG coding by hospitals. In the beginning of the program, PROs did discover improper coding, particularly in small hospitals. This finding related more to the need to upgrade and improve medical record departments than to any conscious efforts to generate higher DRG payments.

In summary, it is still premature to pass judgment on the PRO program. In comparison to PSRO, however, no one disputes that the PRO program represents a significant improvement. The PRO statute and subsequent regulations gave PROs authority to make decisions that PSROs lacked. The advent of PPS created strong political support for PROs that earlier review efforts could not generate. PPS provided the necessary rationale for striking a more appropriate balance between efforts to reduce Medicare program costs and to protect the quality of the care being delivered. The program already appears to be identifying and correcting poor quality care while facilitating more appropriate utilization of services. Most important, the program has moved beyond the question posed by the Reagan Administration: Do we need an external medical review program? The question has now become: How do we improve it?

THE FUTURE CHALLENGE

What are some of the specific challenges ahead for the field of quality assurance in the public sector? Following are some of the issues that need to be addressed if we desire to speak with confidence about the future.

Broadening Access

Quality care begins with access to it. (See Chapter 1.) Many forget that access to care was not guaranteed for all Americans with the passage of Medicare and Medicaid. Solutions to our access problems do exist, however. They include: mandates to employers to provide health benefits, state-mandated insurance risk pools, individual retirement accounts for long-term care coverage, and expanded private and Medicare/Medicaid benefits. The environment, however, is not conducive to such changes. Solutions await a strengthened American economy and some resolution of the federal deficit problem. But thankfully, the access issue, as it was decades ago, is returning as a major national health policy issue.

Ambulatory Review

Reimbursement reforms and other cost containment strategies are driving medical services, technology and personnel to nonacute care settings. Yet, quality assurance activities have focused, almost exclusively, on hospital-based services. Ambulatory review represents the new frontier for medical review, both in terms of quality and utilization. Fortunately, some positive steps have been recently taken to expand review into the ambulatory sector.

Integrated Medical Data Bases

Data represent the lifeblood of any quality assurance effort. Yet, too often, data systems are fragmented and lack completeness and uniformity. Two decades after the establishment of the Medicare program, the databases of Part A and Part B have still not been integrated. It is impossible to track patient utilization and health status indicators over time and across various medical care settings. Only recently did Medicare develop a uniform claim form for inpatient services. The cost-effective monitoring of ambulatory services awaits a uniform data system for outpatient encounters as well.

Outcome Measurement and Research

The ability to judge the efficacy and effectiveness of medical treatment will depend on sound patient outcome measures and the

121

ability to track health status indicators before, during, and after the course of treatment. Did patients do better or worse as a result of the medical treatment? Were the potential benefits of the treatment worth the potential risks and costs? Outcome research and clinical trials will be needed to answer these questions. (See Chapter 2.) Such research would be particularly enriched by the development of meaningful and objective outcome measures. Too often, mortality is the only health status indicator captured in present data sources. Severity-of-illness indices show promise of advancing the measurement outcome, particularly if they are built into present data bases.

Treatment Process Standards

Medical outcome analysis must be related to the actual process of treatment. Can the process explain the negative results? Is there a certain process that can achieve better results than others? Should such a process be made a guide or minimum standard for the therapy? The development of process standards is politically volatile. Physician specialty societies will have to exhibit enlightened leadership to move this issue forward in the best interests of society.

Patient Involvement

Patients will need to become more involved in medical care management in the future. Who but the patient should decide in the uncertain world of medical care whether the benefits of a certain treatment outweigh its potential risks and costs? Is surgery worth the risk of complications? Is it worth the pain and the costs of keeping a loved one on a life-support system when death is imminent? Who but the patient or family member should decide these questions? The failure to invest in medical outcome research has left enormous gaps in our knowledge of the medical risks of alternative therapies. If known, such risks must be communicated directly to the patient to permit informed choices. Finally, patients must be regarded as valuable sources of information on the quality of the treatment they receive. This is particularly true for ambulatory care where little data exist on a routine basis to assess quality.

Release of Data

For years, the medical care industry has argued that the release of complex medical data runs the risk of misinforming the public. A competitive medical marketplace will, however, be dependent upon the availability of information to make informed choices. The demands for meaningful information will intensify in the future. PROs will be viewed as a logical source for much of that information. Already they are required to release hospital-specific data upon request. Learning how to balance the integrity and confidentiality of the peer review process with the legitimate right of the public to know will remain one of the tougher challenges ahead.

Funding

The field of quality assurance will reach maturity only if supported by a sound public and private funding base. Developing the tools of quality assessment and preserving the organizational entities to assure quality will be costly. Present funding levels do not bode well for the future. The PRO budget represents less than one-fifth of 1 percent of the Medicare hospital trust fund. An encouraging sign: Authorization for funding for medical care outcome research was recently enacted into law. It has been poorly budgeted, however.

CONCLUSION

The challenge of assuring quality care in the public sector will not be easily met. Many citizens are left without appropriate access to care. The tools for quality assessment are in the early stages of development. Political support for quality assurance has only been recently realized. Government funding to advance quality assurance activities is scarce in an environment in which the federal deficit dictates national health policy. There are many hopeful signs, however. Quality and access are being increasingly talked about. Many are asking: What are we getting as a result of our investment in medical services? Practice variation data have challenged the medical profession to build a more scientific basis for treatment decisions. The consumer is getting involved and asking whether, and which, treatment benefits outweigh risks. It appears that society is beginning to heed Dr. Ernest A. Codman's half-century-old challenge to monitor the results of medical practice. It will take an increasingly aggressive role by the public sector to see that Dr. Codman's dream is realized.

Chapter 6

Quality Assurance in the Public Sector: The Role of One Peer Review Organization*

Thomas R. Hyngstrom, Ph.D.

At public meetings dealing with quality of care review by Medicare Peer Review Organizations (PROs), the following three questions are frequently asked by physicians:

- Can you define "quality of care?"

- Do you have published standards of care?

- If not, why are you trying to regulate my work?

These rather direct questions are significant in that they speak to larger issues than any one physician's concerns.

First, they are reflective of the tremendous stress now being felt by the medical profession as a whole. For the first time, physicians are being subjected to meaningful external monitoring of their performance. It is of little comfort to them that there is no generally accepted definition of "quality" and that few claim to have specific standards for medical practice. The effective impact both of Medicare's Prospective Payment System (PPS) and HMOs and PPOs in the private sector has been to put individual physicians on notice: "Do not spend one unnecessary dollar in the treatment of your patients but do not make one mistake in the quality of care you deliver."

---

*This chapter focuses on the role of peer review organizations in relation to hospital care. For an exploration of their role with respect to health maintenance organizations and competitive medical plans, see Chapter 9.

These three questions also reflect a general societal concern for the quality of medical care in this country. The federal government's attention to quality is clearly a reaction to a broad public concern. Whether a reality or not, the traditional perception of our health care system has changed since the implementation of the PPS. Prior to PPS, a quest for quality was perceived as driving our system. Financial considerations followed. Today, financial concerns are perceived as the driving force with quality following. While few have presented specific examples of reduced quality of care since the introduction of PPS, many have used such terms as "sicker and quicker" to characterize a perceived reduction in the intensity of services currently being received by Medicare beneficiaries. (See Chapters 5 and 7.)

Finally, the above three questions speak to very basic methodological concerns for those responsibile for ensuring the quality of medical care in the public sector. For instance:

1). How does one undertake to define and measure the quality of health care?

2). How does one do this in the context of governmental bureaucracy: a bureaucracy with prescriptive program guidelines; rapidly changing rules; and actual authority to discipline hospitals and physicians?

3). How does one simultaneously maintain the constructive involvement of hosptials and practitioners as well as the independence of action to discipline specific institutions and individuals?

4). How does one go beyond potentially more satisfying academic understandings of quality to implement changes that will help improve the quality of care being received by one-third of all hospitalized patients?

A number of the chapters of this book have addressed various aspects of these questions. In the remainder of this chapter, I will attempt to respond to them in describing the review functions of the PRO for the state of Illinois, the Crescent Counties Foundation for Medical Care of Naperville, IL.

OVERVIEW

The Historical Background and Organizational Characteristics of the Crescent Counties Foundation for Medical Care

The Crescent Counties Foundation for Medical Care (CCFMC) is the Medicare Utilization and Quality Control Peer Review Organization (PRO) for the state of Illinois. As such, CCFMC is responsible for monitoring the approximately 550,000 acute hospital admissions of Medicare beneficiaries each year to the 240 hospitals in Illinois. For the past three years, CCFMC has also contracted with the Illinois Department of Public Aid to monitor both the utilization of services and the quality of care provided in the state's Medicaid program. Approximately 250,000 individuals are hospitalized annually in this program, 80 percent of these in the city of Chicago.

CCFMC was founded in 1974 as a not-for-profit corporation "to take action to improve health care in Illinois" and provide an organizational vehicle for local physicians to operate the Professional Standards Review Organization (PSRO) in four of the five collar counties surrounding Cook County--hence the name Crescent Counties. (See Chapter 5.) It was one of the eight PSROs in the state of Illinois. In 1984, regulations chartering the PRO program specified that there would be only one PRO entity for each state. After several months of negotiations with the Health Standards and Quality Bureau of the Health Care Financing Administration (HCFA), CCFMC was awarded a two-year, $15.2 million contract for PRO review, starting in November 1984. After a positive evaluation of its performance under this award, a second two-year $15.2 million contract was awarded to CCFMC, to take effect in November 1986. This latter time period is referred to as "the second PRO contract period." (See Chapter 5.)

CCFMC performs PRO review directly in the metropolitan Chicago area and subcontracts review for downstate Illinois to the Central Illinois Medical Review Organization in Champaign-Urbana. More than 3,500 practicing physicians belong to CCFMC or its downstate subcontractor. These members represent approximately 15 percent of all physicians in the state. Of this number, more than 600 regularly perform services for CCFMC either as reviewers, committee members, or technical consultants. All major specialties and subspecialties are represented among these physicians. Physicians performing review are required to be licensed and to have an active practice. They come from a full range of hospital settings--teaching, community, urban, and rural. CCFMC has 200 employees; and its subcontractor, an additional 50. Approximately half of these individuals are registered nurses who, as "review coordinators," perform either utilization or quality review for the PRO.

CCFMC's Board of Directors comprises 23 physicians from across the state, three hospital representatives nominated by the Illinois Hospital Association, and a consumer representative--currently the vice chairman of the Illinois Chapter of the American Association of Retired Persons.

As part of its PRO review function, CCFMC also has extensive data processing and reporting capabilities. Copies of all Illinois Medicare hospital billings are forwarded to it by HCFA. Claims data include patient demographic information, diagnostic and procedure codes and detailed charge data. In addition, we may add review findings.

These claims are maintained in a single data base. They are used to select samples of records for review and for profiling purposes. In addition to a wide variety of reports required by HCFA, each PRO produces reports for the use of its own committees and to report to hospitals. Recent legislation also requires each PRO to release nonidentified profiles to the public on request.

The Representativeness of CCFMC as a PRO

Demographics

In terms of both demographics and overall hospital utiliation, Illinois is, on the whole, representative of the nation at large. Illinois ranks fifth among the states in the size of its Medicare beneficiary population, approximately 1.3 million individuals in 1986. This large number of beneficiaries guarantees a representative mix of diagnostic problems. While the major concentration of the state's hospitals, physicians and hospital admissions are located in, or occur within, the Chicago metropolitan area, fully two-thirds of all hospitals, 40 percent of physicians, and 45 percent of all patient admissions are outside of this metropolitan area. There is thus, in the state, a balanced mix of larger urban hospitals, both community and teaching, as well as rural community hospitals.

Hospital utilization

Prior to the PRO program, Illinois's hospital utilization rates for the Medicare population were in the middle of the range for the nation as a whole. The state's average hospital length of stay was essentially identical to the national average. Longer average lengths of stay, comparable to the northeastern region of the country, could be found in Chicago; while patterns of short stays and higher admission rates common to many of the country's rural areas were present in downstate Illinois.

The first two years of PRO review in Illinois resulted in shifts in utilization that were also typical of other states. For example, the average length of stay for Medicare patients declined by nearly two days and the number of admissions declined by approximately 10 percent from a projected total of 604,000, to approximately 545,000 in 1986. This decline was particularly noteworthy for cases involving surgical procedures capable of being performed on an ambulatory basis. In the specific instance of cataract surgery, for example, the inpatient performance of this procedure declined by 90 percent following the first 18 months of focused PRO review. The cumulative impact of this change was an approximate 15 percent reduction in days of hospitalized care per 1,000 beneficiaries in the state, compared with pre-PRO projections.

Operating philosophy

Although Illinois shares demographic and utiliation characteristics with a number of other states, its approach to PRO review is somewhat individualized. Our approach embodies a philosophy toward review that might be best characterized as "local peer review." This approach has been formally put into operation by the Board of Directors of CCFMC.

For example, a large percentage of our physician and coordinator review is on-site, in the hospitals where the care is actually delivered. In this process, the physician reviewer interacts directly with the attending physician. While more costly and difficult to administer, this review policy is maintained to facilitate communication and face-to-face discussion with the attending physician.

Consistent with policy of "local" review, CCFMC uses as reviewers a large number of practicing physicians from across the state rather than a smaller cadre of full-time reviewers. Few (6 percent) of our physician reviewers consult for more than one day a week, and the average reviewer contributes six hours of work per month. A number of other PROs, by choice or economic necessity, use smaller numbers of physicians and perform more remote review (for example, hospital charts are forwarded to their offices for review).

Finally, CCFMC has expended significant energy and time in balancing its contractual obligation to ensure quality of care with its perceived need to guarantee equity to affected hospitals and physicians. As much time has been spent developing procedures for due process as in developing field review procedures.

This emphasis on due process varies from state to state. For Illinois, it has helped to maintain not only the endorsement of both the state's medical society and hospital association but their active cooperation. This cooperation has facilitated many options for corrective action that might not have been possible otherwise and might not exist in states where a more confrontational relationship exists between the PRO and the provider community.

OUR PRO QUALITY REVIEW PROCESS

CCFMC's review process for quality of care reverses the common notion that a PRO should have explicit standards of quality to which physicians and hospitals are held. Rather than promulgating a single method of treating pneumonia patients, for example, our PRO establishes, through professional consensus, a broad range of treatment plans accepted by most physicians for any one illness. The review system is not designed to train physicians, to teach medicine, or to standardize the practice of medicine among all doctors in the state. It is intended to identify outliers--those physicians who practice medicine in ways not accepted by most of their peers. Joyce Craddick, M.D., has coined the term, "disquality" to describe this approach to defining "what quality is not."[2]

An important characteristic of this approach to review is that it focuses on adverse outcomes. If a patient has not experienced an adverse treatment outcome (whether major or minor) or has not been placed at risk to experience such an outcome, then by definition "disquality" is likely not present. (See Chapter 2.)

A second characteristic of this approach is also important. In addition to noting specific exceptions to the expected outcomes of care, the review process includes the consideration of representative patterns. It is assumed that physicians with an active practice make random errors and are subject to untoward events beyond their control. The PRO review process does not attempt to focus on random errors. However, repeated patterns of minor problems or one or more major problem resulting in significant harm to the patient are closely scrutinized.

Finally, while PRO review is often seen as regulatory and intended to discipline physicians, a broad range of cooperative action is more common in our program. Corrective actions in the form of mandated continuing education, utilization of second opinion programs, mandatory consultations, tutorials, or reduced privileges are frequently used. These actions are seen as particularly appropriate for patterns of problems that can be shown to be subject to correction. Where such corrective action initiatives are not seen as appropriate in the judgment of our physician specialists, a formal sanction process may be initiated. However, the principal objective of our review program is to quickly eliminate any problems uncovered and, therein, any risk to Medicare beneficiaries.

In the PRO program overall, the quality of care review process is divided into three general stages: identification of potential problems; confirmation of actual problems; and then corrective action of, or recommendation to the government for disciplinary actions for, confirmed problems. The first two stages traditionally have been considered local in design and orientation, and they are governed by each PRO's contract with HCFA. The third stage is governed by the more formal rules of the sanction process and falls under the authority of the Office of the Inspector General of the U.S. Department of Health and Human Services.

Problem Identification

For the first two years of the PRO program, quality problems were identified through specific Medical Care Evaluation studies or as an incidental result of the judgment of review coordinators or physicians as they screened records for utilization approval. (See Chapters 2 and 5.) In Illinois, eight MCEs affecting about 10 percent of all Medicare patients were undertaken during this time. These studies evaluated the care of acute myocardial infarction and pneumonia and the necessity of surgery for mastectomy and cholecystectomy.

131

In these studies, our data system selected patient records with the appropriate diagnosis or procedure, and review coordinators then screened these records using fixed criteria. Our review coordinators also applied their nursing judgment to all records being reviewed for reasons such as appropriateness of admission and DRG coding, and noted those in which questionable care appeared to be present.

All records so identified were referred by the coordinators to a physician reviewer during his or her next visit to the hospital. The physician reviewer then reviewed each of these records--independent of any screening criteria. If he or she believed that a possible quality of care issue was present, the record was forwarded out of the hospital to CCFMC's office. This was based on the judgment of the reviewer and not on a published standard of practice. (See Chapter 2.) The reviewer was, in fact, asking, "Would I have treated this patient in this manner?"

During this period, approximately 8 percent of all records screened by a review coordinator were referred to a physician reviewer for possible quality of care problems. Of those, about half (4 percent) were then referred out of the hospital by the physician reviewer. Even though over 8,000 records with potential quality problems were identified in this manner, this process suffered from two weaknesses. The independent identification of records by coordinators proved to be inconsistent in the types and numbers of problems identified (i.e., the reliability of the process was low). (See Chapter 2.) For those records to which medical audit criteria were applied, reliabilty was improved, but since only a small number of charts could be handled in this way, the effect of this more object approach was correspondingly limited.

These weaknesses were addressed in the second PRO scope of work/contract period beginning in the fall of 1986 with the introduction of generic/adverse outcome screens. (See Chapters 2 and 5.) As discussed in Chapter 2, these screens identify adverse outcomes which would not be expected to occur in the optimal care of a hospitalized patient. Using these instruments, one can systematically identify cases with adverse outcomes and that require more in-depth review. The Health Care Financing Administration has required that the PROs use six screens: 1) adequacy of discharge planning; 2) medical stability of patient at discharge; 3) deaths; 4) nosocomial infections; 5) unscheduled return to surgery; and 6) trauma suffered in the hospital. (See Chapter 2.)

These screens are now applied to all the records we review--approximately 30 percent of all Medicare hospital admissions. Using these screens, the reliability of the review process has been substantially increased, insofar as the review coordinator's role is now limited to documenting whether or not an adverse outcome is objectively present. In addition, as stated above, the scope of the review has been expanded to include all records we now review for any reason. Although the long-term efficacy of this system remains to be proven, results from the first year of its use in Illinois suggest that it is more effective in identifying potential quality problems.

Table 1 presents data on rates of generic-screen failure for six months during the first year of screen use in Illinois. During this time, 75,935 cases were reviewed, revealing 21,985 screen failures, for a rate of 29.1 percent. When duplicate failures per patient were removed, failures were noted in 24 percent of the cases. The most frequent screen failure (11.2 percent) was for the screen "medical stability at discharge." Almost 7 percent of the cases failed the nosocomial infection screen; 5.6 percent failed the inhospital trauma screen; and slightly over 3 percent of cases were found to lack adequate discharge planning. The failure rate for the two screens "unscheduled surgery" and "death" were substantially less, 1.5 percent and 0.9 percent respectively.

The physician confirmation rate of these failures varied substantially among the screens. Slightly over 44 percent of the nosocomial infection failures were confirmed by physicians as representing a potential quality problem, but only 8.2 percent of the mortality screen failures were confirmed. The confirmation rate varied among the other screen failures from 37.0 percent for inhospital trauma, to 19.6 percent for medical stability at discharge, to 9.6 percent for unscheduled returns to surgery. A physician reviewer confirmation is not required on the remaining screen, adequacy of discharge planning.

The average rate of confirmation for the five screen categories was 24.1 percent. The magnitude of this rate is influenced by the low rate of confirmation on the "death" and "unscheduled return to surgery" screen. For those remaining, the average rate was 34.2 percent, slightly over a third of the failures on these screens. Overall, the unduplicated confirmation rate was 7 percent of all the cases reviewed.

During the second year, HCFA allowed greater discretion by review coordinators in the elimination of false-positive screen failures. As a result, the unduplicate referral rate now is about 15 percent of the cases reviewed by the coordinators. Of this total, about half (6 to 8 percent) are confirmed by the physician reviewer as representing a potential quality problem. Thus, the use of screens in quality review is currently twice as productive in identifying potential quality problems as the previous system.

Confirmation

In order for one of the potential quality problems identified to be determined to be an actionable quality problem, the case must proceed through a well-defined series of review steps. (See Figure 1.) In this process, multiple committees consisting of numerous physician reviewers must each concur that a shortfall in quality is present. At specific stages in this process, board-certified specialists are utilized and interact directly with the attending physician in question. Although federal guidelines require only a formal warning letter and one meeting with the attending for the determination of a "gross and flagrant violation," we have inserted into our process a number of additional review steps to enhance the due process afforded the attending physician.[3-5]

Following the identification of a potential problem at the local hospital level (Steps 1 and 2 in Figure 1), the patient's medical record is forwarded from the hospital to CCFMC's office. It is then reviewed by a team of two physician reviewers not involved in the original review (Step 3). The function of this "reconsideration panel" is to confirm or deny that a problem exists and, in the case of the latter, to rank the severity of the problem. These physicians are aware that a quality issue has been raised in the case, but they are unaware of the previous findings and act independently and do not communicate with one another. This "blinded" review process was instituted to increase objectivity.

The physicians can rank the seriousness of the quality problem in one of four levels:

Rank I Failure to support by appropriate documentary evidence the medical necessity and quality of the care rendered to the Medicare beneficiary.

Rank II   Medical mishap and/or mismanagement resulting in
           the potential for adverse patient outcome; no detrimen-
           tal effect occurred.

Rank III   Medical mishap and/or mismanagement resulting in
           actual adverse patient outcome requiring additional
           medical and/or surgical treatment.

Rank IV   Medical mishap and/or mismanagement resulting in
           imminent danger of or actual injury to body or mind,
           or death (which otherwise might not have been
           expected to occur).

Ranks I, II, and III are termed "substantial" violations and Rank IV,
a "gross and flagrant" violation. Although Rank III is, by federally
mandated definition, a substantial violation, it is frequently regarded
as potentially as serious as a "gross and flagrant violation" and is
treated as such in our review process.

    If one or both of the physician reviewers believes there is no
problem present, the case is dropped. If both believe that a minor
problem (Rank I or II) is present, but cite different problems, the
case is again dropped. If both physicians concur on the presence
of the same problem and its rank, it is forwarded to the next level
of review. Finally, if the two physicians identify the same problem
but provide a different severity ranking, a third reviewer is typically
used to determine the rank.

    Prior to this point in the review process, there has been no
communication with the attending or with the hospital where the
problem occurred. If a quality problem is confirmed in the above step,
a documentation letter is now sent to the attending physician, summarizing the issue and asking for additional clarification.

    From this point forward, the review process follows one of
two trails, depending on the rank assigned to the issue. (See Figure
1.) Less critical quality issues (Ranks I and II) require only a written
response from the attending physician. This response is reviewed
by a new reconsideration panel, which may accept the attending
physician's explanation and fully reverse the finding of a problem
or downrank the severity of the problem. In such cases, further
action is rarely indicated. The panel may, however, uphold the
previous decision. It may also confirm that a problem did occur,
but that it was the responsibility of an employee or a service of
the hospital and, accordingly, assign it to the hospital. If the

physician chooses not to respond to the panel's request for clarification, the problem is considered confirmed.

For the most part, individual confirmed substantial problems are not further acted upon at this point. Rather, they are accumulated over time and a physician or hospital with multiple, confirmed substantial problems which suggest a pattern may be required to develop a corrective action plan (CAP). The CAP must specify a number of activities and responsibilities, including, among others: 1) the steps to be taken that could reasonably be expected to reduce or eliminate the problem; 2) a time frame for completing the CAP; 3) the individual(s) accountable for its completion; 4) measurable outcomes from the plan; and 5) reporting commitments. After the CAP is developed, it is monitored quarterly for compliance by a subcommittee of the Quality Peer Review Committee. (See Step 5.)

While Rank I or II problems are frequently minor, a continuing pattern of such problems can lead to the next higher level of formal review and to possible sanction development. "Substantial numbers of substantial issues" not resolved by corrective action may be cited as evidence of a physician's "inability and unwillingness" to fulfill his "obligation" to provide health care of acceptable quality.[3] A sanction recommendation may thus be developed even in the absence of more serious "gross and flagrant" violations.

A separate review path is followed by cases assigned a Rank III or Rank IV severity. (See Figure 1.) These potential "gross and flagrant" violations involve significant harm to the patient, the imminent risk of such harm, or death. Federal guidelines suggest that each confirmed gross and flagrant issue must result in a formal warning letter to the attending and a subsequent sanction hearing.[3,4] These same guidelines were also once believed to require the development of a sanction recommendation for a single gross and flagrant case regardless of its representativeness. A number of PROs have acted as such. CCFMC, however, has chosen to elaborate the review process so that a formal warning letter is not issued to the attending physician until the fifth level of review. (See Step 5 in Figure 1.)

For these potential "gross and flagrant" cases, the attending is contacted, requested to submit additional information and invited to meet with a second review panel, the Specialty Subcommittee (Step 4). Unlike the randomly assigned reconsideration panels used for the less serious cases, this panel is mandatorily composed of at least two board certified specialists drawn from the field(s) most pertinent to the quality problem under review. As alluded to above, the attending physician's meeting with this subcommittee is "informal." The step is not required in federal guidelines. We have included it in our local review process as a further safeguard to the attending physician so that potential problems that are not substantiated can be ruled out at this stage without initiating formal sanction procedures.

Following discussion with the attending physician, the Specialty Subcommittee may reverse or downrank the case in question, or uphold the finding of a problem. If upheld, the subcommittee's report is submitted to the next level of review--the Quality Peer Review Committee (QPRC, Step 5). The eight appointed members of this committee consider the findings of the subcommittee. Unless a technical error is found, the QPRC will normally issue a formal warning letter to the attending physician, schedule a sanction hearing, and direct that additional records of the physician be reviewed.

This expanded and intensified review normally involves between 20 and 30 records with attributes (e.g., diagnosis, procedure) similar to the case in question. Its purpose is to establish the representativeness of the case under review. Each record in the sample is reviewed using the same general process already described and presented in Figure 1. This intensified review is expedited and its findings referred to the Sanction Determination Panel (Step 6), which consists of the six physicians on the Executive Committee of the Board of CCFMC. Typically, it meets with the attending physician within 60 to 90 days of the issuance of the formal warning letter. The attending physician is allowed to bring legal counsel and expert witnesses to this formal meeting.

At the meeting, all previous review decisions and the recommendations of the QPRC are considered. Extensive discussion follows opening presentations by a representative of the QPRC and the attending physician. Acting on behalf of CCFMC's Board, the sanction panel considers the merits of each case, verifies that established procedures have been followed, and that due process has been afforded the physician. It also documents the absence of any conflict of interest or capricious or arbitrary decisions by lower level panels. The panel must also rule on both the willingness and ability of each physician being reviewed to correct confirmed problems.

In closed deliberations, the panel may reverse, downrank, or uphold any or all case findings. Secondly, the panel may resubmit the entire case to the QPRC for further review or the initiation of corrective action and monitoring. It may also recommend a sanction action to the full board. No fixed guidelines exist for deciding which cases should result in sanction recommendations. All of CCFMC's recommendations for sanctions, however, have involved multiple gross and flagrant findings.

Should a sanction be recommended, the full Board of Directors, in closed session, reviews a detailed summary of all actions leading to the recommendation (Step 7). Barring the finding of error, the board will then submit a formal sanction recommendation to the Office of the Inspector General of the U.S. Department of Health and Human Services. This recommendation may involve a financial penalty and/or exclusion from participation in the Medicare program for between one and five years.

This outline of CCFMC's quality review process is highly condensed, and yet its key features are clear. The multiple levels of review, involving approximately 40 different physicians, are intended to serve as a safety check against an incorrect or ill-informed decision. As noted by one critic of the federal review program, one, two, or three physicians can make a mistake in judgment, can be careless, or can be prejudiced against another physician. It would be highly unlikely, however, for a great injustice to occur under this process.

The criterion that now emerges is how effectively does this system function? Is there a productive outcome of the review?

Review Outcomes

Frequency of confirmed issues

As stated above, all suspected quality issues are subjected to a multiple-level committee review process with appropriate involvement of the attending physician. During the first two years of PRO review in Illinois, approximately 3,600 quality problems were confirmed through the above process. Of these, 95 percent were Rank I and II problems, 1.8 percent were Rank III, and 4.4 percent were Rank IV. The overwhelming majority (95 percent) of the above cases involved an individual physician rather than a hospital.

As of December 1987, CCFMC has recommended four physicians and one hospital for sanction to the Office of the Inspector General.

Approximately three dozen additional cases from the first two years of review have sanction hearings pending. An equal number of physicians with confirmed Rank III cases have been placed on intensified review and ongoing monitoring. Finally, 57 of the 100 hospitals in the Chicago metropolitan area are being required to develop corrective action plans to address patterns of substantial quality issues identified in their physician staffs.

Table 2 presents a summary of the review outcomes for cases initially assigned a Rank IV in Step 3 of our process. The specific records cited are the first 56 of approximately 150 such cases. The remaining cases have yet to complete all steps of the review process. Preliminary analysis of their status, however, suggests the same distribution is likely. As can be seen, almost one half of these cases were confirmed as Rank IV. Slightly over half of the remaining were downranked, and the remainder reversed, requiring no further action.

Slightly over half of the confirmed cases resulted in intensified monitoring or the establishment of a CAP. Almost a quarter of the cases were set aside owing to the retirement of the physician involved. Four of the cases were reassigned from the attending to the hospital and a CAP requested. Examples of cases in this category include inadequate supervision of medical students in the care of patients, and inadequate performance of hospital ancillary services, particularly with regard to timely communication with, and support of, the attending physician. The CAPs to be developed in these instances will address these deficiences in care and propose steps to eliminate them.

Only two of the 27 confirmed Rank IV cases resulted in a referral to the Sanction Determination Panel for a sanction recommendation. Thus, one can see that sanctioning for the sake of sanctioning is not one of our goals. We are interested in finding the most appropriate corrective action to assure that the quality of care being delivered to Medicare beneficiaries is enhanced to the maximum extent possible.

As noted earlier, the use of generic adverse outcome screens in the last two years has doubled our rate of problem identification. However, the second scope of work simultaneously reduced the total volume of cases required to be reviewed by PROs from approximately 45 percent of all Medicare admissions to approximately 30 percent. Thus, the net result of these two changes is expected to be a slight increase in the number of problems identified and ultimately confirmed through our process.

Characteristics of confirmed issues

Table 3 is an array by diagnosis of the most common categories of quality problems for a sample of 68 recently tabulated Rank IV cases. As can be seen, general medical conditions such as myocardial infarction, heart failure and chest pain predominate, as opposed to surgical problems or trauma. The bulk of the problems are in the category of incomplete or improper diagnostic work-up, testing, or monitoring, followed by errors in care and follow-up. Table 4 provides specific examples of the types of quality problems found in a number of the categories given in Table 3.

The specific examples presented in Table 4 were rated as Rank IV problems because of the harm that resulted to the patient in the specific case. It is not uncommon, however, for some of these same types of quality problems to be rated as Rank I or Rank II violations where the level of harm resulting to the patient is potential or minor. For instance, we have found that up to one-fourth of the confirmed Rank I and II problems at large urban hospitals involve incomplete or inconsistent monitoring of patients with apparent heart problems. The vast majority of these incidents do not result in any harm to the patient. The frequency of this same problem in Rank IV cases, however, makes it advisable that we address monitoring in our corrective actions. Thus, on the basis of our findings, a number of the above hospitals have been required to develop CAPs for monitoring. Typically, such patterns of substantial problems involve many different physicians, most of whom may have only one confirmed case. Thus, to address the problem adequately, the hospital is asked to implement corrective programs that will impact on all their physicians.

Distribution of problems by provider

CCFMC's experience has been that quality problems are distributed widely throughout the patient population. They are not evenly distributed, however. Figures 2 and 3 display the distribution of confirmed substantial issues by hospital and physician in the Chicago metropolitan area for 1986-87.

These figures show a large number of hospitals and physicians with a small number of problems. Eventually, most physicians will probably receive at least one initial documentation letter or confirmation of a minor quality issue. The critical finding from the figures, however, is the concentration of problems in a few hospitals and a few physicians. Specifically, 6 percent of the hospitals have 20 percent of the problems, and 4 percent of the physicians have 15 percent of them. Graphs for initial generic screen failures and quality issues identified through our Medicaid review program also show the same phenomenon. Hospitals or physicians with extreme scores on any one of these graphs tend to have extreme scores on several.

CCFMC interprets these findings as supporting the notion that virtually all hospitals and physicians have occasional random quality problems, but a small number of each is evidence of a consistent pattern of such problems. Althouhg limited, this small percentage of hospitals and physicians with multiple issues treat thousands of patients yearly. Identifying them would appear to be a major positive outcome of our review process. Modifying their practice patterns should be of immediate benefit to the patients they treat.

CONCLUSION

Our data suggest that the overall quality of care received by Medicare beneficiaries in Illinois is high. Approximately 98 percent of the cases reviewed are determined to have received care consistent with generally accepted medical standards. The results from PROs in other states suggest similar findings. (See Chapter 5.) Our review process appears to be able to detect deficiencies in care and in a way that preserves the "due process" of the providers involved. Its ability to identify providers with patterns of repeated quality problems suggests an ability to reach those providers most in need of corrective action. Similarly, our broadly based, hospital CAPs have the potential of general improvements in the quality of care for large numbers of patients.

CCFMC believes that its approach to quality review--one which emphasizes the positive aspects of improving the quality of care, avoids unnecessarily harsh penalties, and regularly involves thousands of physicians in private review of their work--is and will continue to be productive in accomplishing the PRO mission of safeguarding and enhancing the quality of care of Medicare beneficiaries--and indirectly the quality of care of all Americans.

Figure 1. PRO quality review and sanction process.

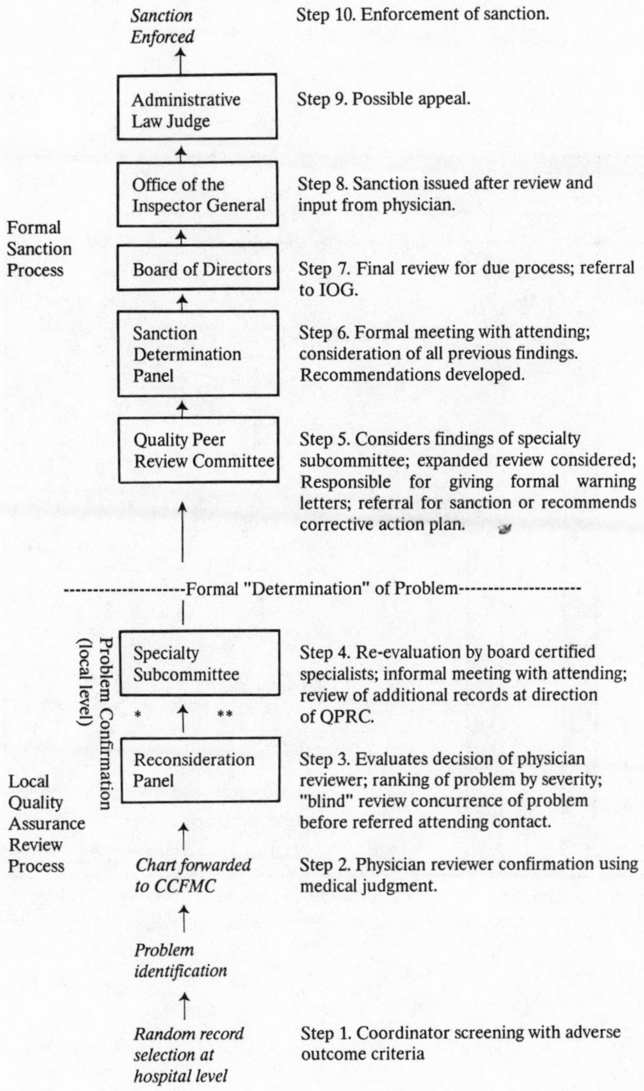
Sanction Enforced
Step 10. Enforcement of sanction.
Administrative Law Judge
Step 9. Possible appeal.
Office of the Inspector General
Step 8. Sanction issued after review and input from physician.
Formal Sanction Process
Board of Directors
Step 7. Final review for due process; referral to IOG.
Sanction Determination Panel
Step 6. Formal meeting with attending; consideration of all previous findings. Recommendations developed.
Quality Peer Review Committee
Step 5. Considers findings of specialty subcommittee; expanded review considered; Responsible for giving formal warning letters; referral for sanction or recommends corrective action plan.
Formal "Determination" of Problem
Problem Confirmation (local level)
Specialty Subcommittee
Step 4. Re-evaluation by board certified specialists; informal meeting with attending; review of additional records at direction of QPRC.
*
**
Reconsideration Panel
Step 3. Evaluates decision of physician reviewer; ranking of problem by severity; "blind" review concurrence of problem before referred attending contact.
Local Quality Assurance Review Process
Chart forwarded to CCFMC
Step 2. Physician reviewer confirmation using medical judgment.
Problem identification
Random record selection at hospital level
Step 1. Coordinator screening with adverse outcome criteria

*Rank III or IV case goes to specialty subcommittee.
**Rank I or II case gets written response from attending physician and is referred back to Sanction Reconsideration Panel.

Figure 2. Hospitals with confirmed substantial problems (1986-1987).

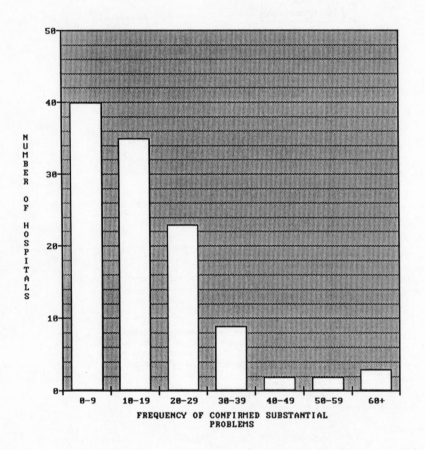

Figure 3. Frequency distribution of confirmed substantial problems by hospitals in Chicago metropolitan area, 1986-1987.

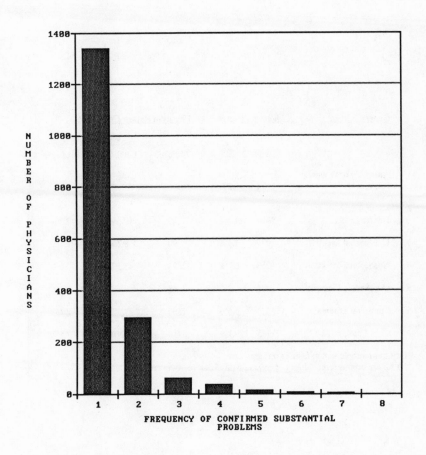

Table 1

Failure Rates for Adverse Outcome Generic Screens in PRO Quality Review In Illinois

(N = 75,935 Reviews)

	Generic Screen	Screen Failures		Physician Review Confirmed		
		Number*	%	Number	% of Screen Failures	% of All Cases Screened
1.	Adequacy of Discharge Planning**	2394	3.2%	N/A**		
2.	Medical Stability at Discharge	8494	11.2%	1667	19.6%	2.2%
3.	Unexpected Death	1099	1.5%	90	8.2%	.1%
4.	Nosocomial Infection	5058	6.7%	2293	45.3%	3.0%
5.	Unscheduled Surgery	706	.9%	68	9.6%	.1%
6.	Inhospital Trauma	4234	5.6%	1600	37.8%	2.1%
	Total:	21985	29.1%	5718	NA	7.5%

*Includes multiple screen failures on same case.
**A failure on this screen does not require a physician reviewer confirmation.

Table 2

Specific Review Outcomes
for the First 56 Cases Assigned a "Rank IV"
in Step 3 of our Review Process

		Number	Percent
1.	Confirmed as Rank IV Cases and Action Taken	27	48
A.	Intensified monitoring; either sanction or corrective action is still possible	8	14
B.	Established corrective action plans	7	12
C.	Retirement of physicians with confirmed cases set aside; no further action required	6	11
D.	Responsibility for case reassigned from attending to the hospital; correction action plan to be developed	4	7
E.	Referred to Sanction Determination Panel for sanction recommendation	2	4
2.	Case Downranked		
	Subject to corrective action if patterns are present	16	29
3.	Reversed		
	No further action	13	23
	Total:	56	100

Table 3

Characteristics of Confirmed Rank IV Cases
By Diagnosis and Category of Quality Problem

(N = 68)

		Category of Quality Problem		
Diagnosis	Number of Case/%	Incomplete/ Improper Diagnosis	Incomplete/ Improper Diagnostic Work-up, Testing, Monitoring	Improper Care, Medication, Surgical Technique	Inadequate Follow-up Premature Discharge, or Unstable Transfers
Myocardial infarction/ chronic heart failure	19 (28%)	3	16	3	4
Chest pain	15 (22%)	1	11	1	1
Pneumonia	8 (12%)	--	5	5	3
Arrhythmia/angina	6 (9%)	--	3	1	--
Abdominal pain	5 (7%)	--	3	2	1
Diabetes	2 (3%)	--	2	--	1
Cerebral vascular accident	2 (3%)	--	2	1	--
Other	11 (16%)	1	7	3	3
Totals:	68 (100%)	5 (6%)	49 (59%)	16 (19%)	13 (16%)

Table 4

Specific Examples of Confirmed Rank IV Quality Problems By Category of Problem

1. Incomplete Work-up or Testing

   ▪ Lack of treatment for noted symptoms.

   Example: Patient required admission for congestive heart failure and dyspnea. Physical findings on admission revealed "left leg swollen, red, and has a positive squeeze reflex on the calf." No diagnostic tests or anticoagulants were ordered for these findings.

   ▪ Inadequate work-up.

   Example: Patient was admitted with abdominal pain and hematemesis, increasing dyspnea. Patient has history of massive cardiomegaly and early congestive heart failure, which was not addressed in record. No CBC on admission.

   ▪ No repeat of abnormal tests.

   Example: Patient admitted for cataract surgery; potassium level was 3.0 on admission and dropped to 2.5 post operatively. No repeat lab test and no follow-up ordered. No treatment or documentation noted in medical record.

2. Improper Care

   ▪ Patients admitted with possible cardiac symptoms.

   ▪ Most common problem -- patient was not admitted to a monitored unit when presented to the hospital with symptoms of possible cardiac involvement.

Table 4, continued

Example: Following a near syncopal episode with a diagnosis of aortic stenosis and sinus bradycardia, with pulse rate of 44, documented in the emergency room, patient was admitted to hospital but not to a monitored unit.

3. Premature Discharge

Example: Patient was admitted for incarcerated hernia; had emergency repair and bowel resection. At time of discharge patient had a low grade fever and tender groin. He was readmitted six days later with an inguinal abscess.

4. Inappropriate Transfers

■ No documentation as to reason for transfer or patient not medically stable when transferred.

Example: Patient was transferred from an acute hospital to a rehabilitation unit with an active pulmonary disease. Temperature 101.2 degrees, and the chest X-rays showed infiltrates and pleural effusion on admission to the rehabilitation unit.

NOTES

1. Health Care Financing Administration, Office of Professional Standards Review Organizations, *PHDDS Report Series,* May 1982.

2. J.W. Craddick, "The Medical Management Analysis System," *Quality Review Bulletin,* April (1979): 2-8.

3. Health Care Financing Administration, *Peer Review Organization Manual* (transmittal no. 5) (Rockville, MD: Department of Health and Human Services, August 1985).

4. Health Care Financing Administration, *Peer Review Organization Manual* (transmittal no. 6) (Rockville, MD: Department of Health and Human Services, October 1985).

5. Health Care Financing Administration, *Peer Review Organization Manual* (transmittal no. 15) (Rockville, MD: Department of Health and Human Services, May 1987).

Chapter 7

The Emergence of Quality of Care Issues in Medicare and How to Address Them: A Consumer Perspective

Jack E. Christy, J.D.

Medicare's new prospective payment system (PPS) for hospitals dramatically changed the way in which hospitals are paid for providing care to the elderly and the disabled. As a result, hospitals now face strong incentives to limit both the length of stay and the intensity of care for their Medicare patients.

Hospitals had a strong and early response to the incentives in the new system. During its first year, the length of stay for Medicare beneficiaries fell by 9 percent. Interestingly, Medicare admissions also fell by 4 percent in that year, the first decline since the program was initiated. Hospitals reduced expenses by laying off staff, eliminating beds, and negotiating lower prices with suppliers. The use of expensive inpatient procedures was curbed. A study by the General Accounting Office (GAO), for example, found that the use of intensive care units by Medicare patients was also lower.[1] GAO attributed this response to the incentives in PPS. Similarly, the Commission on Professional and Hospital Activities found that the use of cardiac care units also declined during the first year of PPS.[2]

PPS also encourages hospitals to limit the inpatient stay to those services necessary to stabilize the patient's condition. Patients who need recuperative care or care requiring less intensive medical supervision are generally now discharged to skilled nursing facilities or home settings. The tail end of the hospital stay for a recuperating, frail, 85-year-old patient with limited abilities, which most likely would have been paid for under the traditional cost-based reimbursement system, is no longer considered part of the inpatient stay. Hospitals no longer permit patients to remain hospitalized until a suitable skilled nursing bed is available. Under the old cost-based system, these "administratively necessary days" (ANDs) were reimbursed by Medicare. Owing to the way the DRG payments were calculated, the monies previously paid for these ANDs were included

153

in the determination of the level of DRG payment for each hospitalization and are therein made available to the hospital. The ANDs are no longer available, however, to patients awaiting placement in appropriate post-hospital settings.

Although on paper the Medicare program offers home health care and skilled nursing services for persons needing post-hospital care, these services are often not available. Early trends indicate that use of these two services, which together account for less than 3 percent of all Medicare spending, has not grown in response to quicker hospital discharges and shorter lengths of stay. In home health care alone, the average annual spending growth rate of 25 percent, seen each year between 1981 and 1984, fell to 15 percent in 1985.

Utilization data show a similiar trend. According to the Health Care Financing Administration (HCFA), the increase in home health visits in 1984 was less than any year-to-year increase since the Omnibus Budget Reconciliation Act of 1980.[4] Moreover, Medicare-covered days per 1,000 enrollees for skilled nursing care have declined steadily since 1977.[5] Thus, patients faced with a tightening of health care resources and consequent cutbacks in care are questioning, and rightly so, just what is being bought with their health care dollars.

The American Association of Retired Persons believes that the answer to this question must come from the development of a quality-of-care assessment and assurance system that identifies quality of care problems in a timely way and implements appropriate corrective actions. Such a system does not now exist, but it can be developed. Whether it will be developed depends to a large extent on the level of national concern over the erosion of health care benefits in the 1980s.

DEFINING A QUALITY HEALTH CARE "BUY"

Our nation's ability to better assure high quality medical care is directly related to: 1) our understanding of what a quality medical outcome is; and 2) our ability to promptly detect and correct unacceptable deviations from quality care. The fact of the matter is, however, our country lacks adequate information about medical outcomes and the quality monitoring system necessary to promptly alert providers and policymakers to unacceptable care.

Fortunately, for most workers with health insurance coverage and Medicare beneficiaries, receiving poor quality medical care is the exception rather than the rule. Systemic lapses in the quality of care found in some underfunded Medicaid, county, and state programs continue to be overlooked mainly because the constituents of such programs are politically weak. Medicare beneficiaries, on the other hand, are perceived to be politically strong.

Until PPS, quality of care was not much of an issue in Medicare. It is startling to discover that the word "quality" does not even appear in the Medicare statute, Title XVIII of the Social Security Act. Prior to PPS, an apparent abundance of resources helped camouflage issues concerning the quality of services under Medicare. Fiscal intermediaries (FIs) and carriers, the administrators of Medicare claims, have no designated functions concerning the quality of care provided to beneficiaries. Few FIs or carriers collect data in a uniform way and thus have limited abilities to compare and contrast data and trends. As a result, there is very little hard data about the quality of the medical services provided under Medicare. One of the goals of the Peer Review Organization (PRO) Program is to develop such data.

To improve the measuring of various dimensions of quality of medical care, priority must be given to the development of monitoring and reporting systems specifically devoted to quality. Progress in developing such a system, however, has been hampered by the problem of defining quality of health care. Traditionally, quality of care has been thought of as a multidimensional construct encompassing structure, process, and outcomes of care, any or all of which may be viewed as particularly important in different contexts.

Unfortunately, there is no definition of quality of medical care that states how the different dimensions of quality--structure, process, outcome--should be combined in an overall assessment of quality. (See Chapter 1 for an approach to formulating an overall assessment.) Each of these dimensions provides different types of information. Each dimension permits different levels of direct involvement and control by providers, patients, third-party payers, and regulators. Thus, a comprehensive definition of quality of medical care is stalled by both technical problems related to limitations of information and methodologies for producing valid measures, and by political and economic problems related to the purpose of the assessment process itself and who should be involved in it.

AN EMERGING NEW ERA IN QUALITY ASSURANCE?

The interest in quality health care initiated by PPS is nourishing a new era in quality assessment. This new era seeks to identify poor-quality performance and outcomes by focusing on statistically aberrant performances or outcomes.

HCFA helped to further open the door to statistically based quality analysis by publishing hospital-specific mortality data in 1986 and 1987[6]. This is especially true of the 1987 disclosure which was planned and executed with much greater care than the first disclosure in 1986. Although disclosure of provider-specific data is still in the development phase, and legitimate questions can be raised about aspects of both HCFA disclosures (see Chapters 1 and 2), they have helped to establish review of statistically aberrant providers as a useful way to assess quality in medical care. They have also shown a strong correlation between the volume of procedures performed in an institution and the outcomes of those procedures. (See Chapter 2.)

In addition, Dr. John Wennberg's landmark research on small area variations and health care practice styles and costs has demonstrated that similiar health outcomes among patient populations matched by age, sex, and race are possible over a wide range of utilization rates.[7] A major step in understanding the outcomes of care is to understand the variations in the provision of care. Only after the variations in the practice of medicine are understood will the degree to which health care is clinically appropriate in a given circumstance be understood and lead to the development of clear quality standards. (See Chapter 8.) The 1986 budget act requires HCFA to document practice variations in at least twelve states and calls for studying patient outcomes for selected diagnoses. PROs in the selected states are expected to be the focal point for this important new initiative.[8]

QUALITY ASSURANCE IN MEDICARE

PROs are private entities that contract with HCFA to review utilization and quality of services under Medicare's PPS. (See Chapters 5 and 6.) PROs have a crucial role in assuring that high-quality medical care is maintained in Medicare and, thus, have important responsibilities with regard to the development of a national quality monitoring system.   As greater and greater cost efficiencies are squeezed out of PPS, the PROs' role as guardians of quality in Medicare services becomes even more important.   PROs must be leaders in the development of innovative methods for tracking various dimensions of quality and in translating that information so that it is useful to health care consumers.

PROs are government contractors, however, and, as such, must implement federal policies. By their nature, PROs reflect and represent federal policies. By their nature, PROs also reflect and represent professional and provider perspectives.   At the same time, not withstanding all these pressures and dynamics, Medicare beneficiaries look to PROs to act as the allies and the   advocates for the patient community.   Ultimately, the success of PROs will depend upon putting patients' interests first.   This priority entails implementing a review strategy that truly improves health outcomes while respecting the physician-patient bonds that attend the healing process, bonds that have come under severe strain in recent years.   It is in the interest of both patients and PROs to maintain an efficient, cost-effective health care system that at the same time remains humane, caring, and capable of renewing the trust and mutual respect between doctor and patient that is critical to patients' recovery from illness.

PROs have a central role to play in assuring quality in Medicare. The myriad problems inherent in establishing a nationwide utilization and quality monitoring and assurance program have slowed the full realization of their role, however.   Moreover, the Omnibus Budget Reconciliation Act of 1987 eroded PROs' authority to sanction practitioners providing poor quality care, thus diluting the PROs' ability to meet their statutory obligation to safeguard the quality of care under Medicare.[9]

Continuing medical price inflation and large federal deficits looming in the fiscal years ahead mean that Medicare will continue to be under intense pressure to cut costs. Quality of care could be the casualty in that process. To maintain quality in Medicare under such relentless pressures will require an even more aggressive and sophisticated system of peer review than is now available.

For peer review to operate in the public's best interest, two essential elements must animate the PRO program.   First, a basic quality assurance program must assure quality from one setting to another.   The 1986 budget act added significant authority to the

157

PROs' mandate for a comprehensive review system. In addition, the new law's requirements for discharge planning, coupled with PROs' increasing application of generic quality screens, give the promise of added protections against one of the problems induced by PPS-- the incentive to discharge patients too soon in their recovery period.

Quality issues are not limited to the inpatient setting. The current reductions in length of hospital stay, increases in patient transfers, and greater use of outpatient services all point to the need for studying quality and the outcomes of care after hospital discharge. Beyond requiring PROs to review care in the ambulatory and post-acute care settings, understanding the broader effects of PPS will require studies of an entire episode of illness from diagnosis and treatment through recovery, regardless of the site of care. The mechanisms to be used by PROs in their review of health maintenance organizations participating in Medicare provide an example of the growing awareness of the need to think in terms of entire episodes of illness. (See Chapter 9.)

Second, in connection with the critical role of data in quality assurance, there is an overriding need for PROs to develop and make available analyzed, comparative data and information about the outcomes and implications of their review responsibilities. The debate about data disclosure has shifted from a focus on whether information should be published at all, to how to release data so consumers can use it effectively. PROs must rise to the challenge of turning raw statistics into a picture patients can understand. Toward that end, the PROs' role as analyzer and disseminator of data will become ever more crucial to their future success.

The dissemination of information is not the PROs responsibility alone. HCFA is accountable publically for data disclosure, too. There are several things HCFA could do to help inform health care consumers about buying health care services. For example, efforts to link data from Part A and Part B of Medicare, which is necessary for reviewing an entire episode of illness, must proceed as a high priority project. Physicians should be required to include uniformly coded diagnosis data on Part B claims. Diagnosis information is important for measuring and monitoring quality in various settings of care. High priority should be given to the development of patient-oriented quality assessment in post-hospital care, such as skilled nursing facilities and home health care. (See Chapter 11.)

Constructing such a quality assessment and assurance system will require much greater coordination among the HCFA contractors administering Medicare. Intermediaries, carriers, and PROs must begin to collect and process basic data elements in a uniform way so that there is comparability among providers. Standardization of quality of care measures and methodologies will give greater assurance to beneficaries about the quality of their medical care and lead to nationally representative data.

The information collected by this quality assessment and assurance system should serve as the basis for a national epidemiological data base of relevant patient-level data on the overall quality of care to Medicare patients, regardless of the setting of care. Such a data base will be an invaluable tool for assessing beneficaries' access to the various levels of care and will lead to greater understanding of the ways in which quality affects beneficaries' health status and quality of life.

DATA DISCLOSURE: THE HERE AND NOW

Several available measures related to PRO review currently would yield information of value, not just to Medicare beneficaries but to the development of a comprehensive quality-of-care assurance system for all. Subject both to maintaining strict patient confidentiality and the development of reporting formats, PROs, on a routine basis, should collect, analyze, and translate for consumers usable, provider-specific information. For example, PROs could profile all cases of denials of care, all patients required to obtain services as an outpatient, and all patient complaints by provider. In addition, a standardized methodology for determining a valid nosocomial infection rate by provider would give consumers a very useful piece of information. Routine reports on the number of readmissions resulting from premature discharge or lack of post-acute care services occurring within thirty to sixty days of discharge, by provider, would give health care consumers important information about the operation of the Medicare program.

DATA DISCLOSURE: OVER THE LONG TERM

Over the longer term, new data elements must be incorporated into the system so that quality is understood through the continuum of care (ambulatory through custodial), and instances of poor quality are detected and corrected promptly, regardless of the setting of care. The quality-of-care data elements to be developed over the longer term include: 1) improved measures that describe the severity of illness and the functional status of patients; 2) the development of valid and comparable measures for quality in ambulatory care, skilled nursing care, and home health care; and 3) the profiling of cases of PROs denying reimbursement under their authority to deny payment for poor-quality care.

CONCLUSION

It is possible to assess the quality of health care services by considering both population-based rates of utilization resulting from small-area analysis of physician practice patterns and primary clinical data, such as laboratory test results and physical findings from the patient's medical chart to help determine the efficiency, effectiveness, and appropriateness of the care--the quality of care--being delivered. The combination of both small-area analysis and clinical effectiveness data provide assessment of both macro- and micro-level performance by providers.

The challenge is to develop such indicators into a coherent system of quality assurance from setting to setting and to translate such data into information useful to consumers. Health care consumers in general, and Medicare beneficiaries in particular, have an important stake in developing a reliable, independent, health care information system. Medical price inflation will continue to put pressure on all third-party payers, both public and private, to cut costs. It will take all the resolve that consumers can muster to overcome, in an era of strict cost containment, the powerful institutional forces against the implementation of a health care information and quality monitoring system. Without such a system, however, the quality of care for too many Americans could drop below acceptable standards. The routine publication of information useful to consumers will assure that health care providers compete on the basis of quality and that the dynamics of the system will help enforce high standards of care.

NOTES

1. "Past Overuse of Intensive Care Services Inflates Hospital Payment" (GAO/HRD-86-25) (Washington, DC: General Accounting Office, March 1986).

2. "The Impact of the Prospective Payment System on the Quality of Care" (Ann Arbor, MI: Commission on Professional and Hospital Activities, November 1985).

3. S. Leader, "Home Health Care Benefits Under Medicare" (AARP Public Policy Institute Issue Brief #8601) (Washington, DC: American Association of Retired Persons, 1986).

4. W. Callahan, "Medicare Use of Home Health Services" *Health Care Financing Review,* 7(1985): 89.

5. Unpublished tables from the Health Care Financing Administration, Karen Beebe, Statistical Information Services Branch, September 1986.

6. "Medicare Hospital Mortality Information" (Rockville, MD: U.S. Department of Health and Human Services, Health Care Financing Administration, December 1987).

7. J. Wennberg and A. Gittelsohn, "Variations in Medicare Care Among Small Areas," *Scientific American,* (April 1982).

8. "AMRRC Negotiates with HCFA to Conduct Small-Area Analysis Educational Project," *Quality Review News,* 2(Fall 1987).

9. Section 4095, "Preexclusion Hearings," Omnibus Budget Reconciliation Act of 1987, December 12, 1987.

Chapter 8

Enhancing Quality Through
Small Area Analysis: The Maine Experience

Robert B. Keller, M.D.

In the post-World War II era, "quality" of care became something of a given in medical practice in the United States. Without concern for cost, physicians and the health care establishment focused their considerable energies on this concept. While "quality" was not in any way measured, it was felt that more was better. As a result, we produced more hospitals, more physicians, and more technology, believing that quality of care would inevitably follow. What also followed was an unplanned, and apparently unacceptable, increase in cost. This has triggered major concerns among all levels of payers, from individual patients to the federal government. While methods that attempt to control costs are legion, the idea of pure cost control is not appealing to physicians and presents political problems to those who would regulate care. As tax payers, we would like to spend less on medical care, but as individual patients, we tend to be more concerned about quality than cost.

The question then remains: how can we control the costs of medical care and simultaneously preserve quality of care? We are faced with the problem of spending less and preserving quality in a health care system which has the highest utilization in the world. A partial answer to this quandry can be found in the concept of small-area analysis. Developed by Wennberg and Gittlesohn, this methodology focuses on the study of variations in physician practice patterns.[1]

METHODOLOGY

In the small-area analysis concept, patients are grouped into hospital service areas centered around medical facilities where the majority of the population receives its care. These areas are con-structed through the use of statewide hospital discharge data bases and are adjusted for age, sex, and so on. Analysis of geographically based population data gives a more accurate measure of distribution of medical services than either hospital-based or physician-based data. The "actual" rates for medical and surgical treatment can be calculated for each area and compared to state and national rates. Actual rates are then compared to "expected" rates. Expected rates are calculated for each hospital service area by applying the average statewide rate to the area under study.

Dr. John Wennberg has found that for diagnoses and procedures where there is consensus among physicians regarding appropriate methods of treatment, rates of care vary very little.[2] Examples of nonvariable conditions include admission for myocardial infarction, treatment of hip fracture, and herniorrhaphy. Conversely, when physician consensus is lacking, rates may vary widely for procedures such as hysterectomy, tonsillectomy, and surgery for disc herniation, and for admissions for such conditions as pneumonia and gastro-intestinal diseases. These latter conditions are dubbed "variable." The difference between high and low rates of admission results in thousands of hospitalizations and a massive expenditure of funds. If analysis demonstrates that high rates of admission and treatment are not necessary, and physicians can lower those rates, large amounts of money can be saved and quality of care enhanced.

THE MAINE MEDICAL ASSESSMENT PROGRAM

The Maine Medical Assessment Program (MMAP) is based on the small-area analysis concept.[3] In 1978, Maine began to collect total hospital discharge data. Because of the quality of these data, Wennberg began to study variations in the state. With the interest and support of Dr. Daniel F. Hanley, then editor of *The Journal of the Maine Medical Association,* MMAP was established in 1980 under the leadership of Hanley and Wennberg. Initially, physicians in Maine as a whole, as well as the leadership of the Maine Medical Association, expressed considerable reservation about the project. This concern was based on a distrust of the validity of the data, concern about inappropriate use of the information, and concern over public exposure of doctors.

Time and experience have now convinced almost all Maine physicians of the value of MMAP. The medical association now is a strong supporter and acts as fiscal intermediary for grant monies.

MMAP is directed by Dr. Hanley and an advisory committee composed of Maine-based health care professionals and academic consultants such as Wennberg. It has received funding from the Commonwealth Fund, the Robert Wood Johnson Foundation, the Bingham Fund, and Maine Blue Cross/Blue Shield.

Within MMAP, there are seven specialty study groups: internal medicine, pediatrics, family practice, obstetrics/gynecology, urology, orthopedics, and ophthalmology. The study group leaders are respected, clinicians practicing in their specialty. It has been found that orientation to specialty groups has been much more successful than attempting to present data to heterogeneous physician groups such as medical staffs, county medical societies, and so on. Groups of specialists appear to understand better the significance of specific variations and are comfortable in openly discussing them and making recommendations to their peers.

Data for the MMAP study groups are processed by the Maine Health Information Center (MHIC), an independent research organization. MHIC receives copies of the total hospital discharge data files from the state and formulates reports for MMAP. The overall data file is public information under state supervision, but specific reports and projects done for MMAP are held confidentially within the project.

STUDY GROUPS

Study groups target diagnoses and procedures in their specialty which exhibit significant variation. Using the hospital discharge data file, ICDA-9 codes are carefully refined so that statistical information is precise and accurate. Each study group must learn the basic concepts of small-area analysis and be convinced of the validity of both the approach and the data. Study group meetings are held in a confidential, educational format with participants from high-, middle-, and low-rate areas. If high rates of medical care are not supportable, the effects of peer pressure are readily apparent. We call this process "feedback," and it is almost always effective in influencing rates. We have learned that, first, physicians do not know the rates at which they practice; and, second, they are uncomfortable as "statistical outliers." Once convinced of the validity of the data, and lacking any peer support, a prompt decrease in high rates of medical care has been the rule.

MMAP's orthopedic study group has focused on surgery for herniated intervertebral disc, a variable procedure in Maine and across the country. Figure 1 illustrates the extent of variation and shows that, in 1984, Maine had very high laminectomy rates, compared with the rest of the country. The workers' compensation subgroup was studied extensively, because historically this group of patients has responded less well to surgery than the general population.[4] While minor variations existed within the state from 1980 to 1982, overall rates began to rise rapidly from 1983 to 1984 (Figure 2). Analysis of small-area data revealed that the majority of the increase in procedures was occuring in one area consisting of a city and three adjacent communities. Surgical rates in these areas prior to 1983 had been below the state average, but increased sharply from 1983 to 1984 (Figure 3). Further study showed that essentially all operations were being performed in the urban area, even though surgeons qualified to perform the procedures practiced in all four areas. Careful study of potential causes for the rate change suggested an increase in physician manpower in the urban community as the explanation.

Thus, early in 1985, the orthopedic study group met with orthopedists and neurosurgeons from the targeted area. Vigorous discussion indicated that physician peers did not feel that the high surgical rates were appropriate. The "feedback" process occured. As indicated in Figure 2 and Figure 3, rates of surgery decreased to the state average over the next one and one-half years.

Hospitalization for treatment of common pediatric illnesses such as pneumonitis and gastroenteritis is discretionary, and rates of admission are variable. Figure 4 presents the number of admissions for four pediatric conditions in one Maine city compared with the expected number based on the state average. In the early 1980s, those admissions were 2.4 times higher than the other city. When the chief of pediatrics in the high-rate area became aware of the data, he began a simple feedback process which involved the public posting of each physician's admissions on a monthly basis. As shown in the figure, rates dropped significantly. When the service chief retired in 1984, rates began to rise again. Feedback was then provided by the pediatric study group, and rates have declined a second time. This example illustrates that the constantly changing medical climate can result in rising rates after apparent resolution of a problem and that variation data must be monitored on a continuing basis. The positive responses to both instances of feedback in this example also suggest that the reduction in rates associated with feedback is more than an observation of the phenomenon known as "regression to the mean."

OUTCOME STUDIES

While the approach varies, each study group has been successful in dealing with problems of practice variation and has been able to accomplish this task on a voluntary, cooperative basis. Unlike many programs that attempt to influence behavior, MMAP has been able to maintain the support of physicians and has grown in acceptance and stature in Maine and beyond. The program has been recognized by the American Medical Association and has been presented at many national and international meetings.[3] We believe this positive response has occurred because the program is run by practicing physicians, analyzes utilization data in an appropriate way, and engages the medical community in a nonthreatening, educational process that encourages cooperation rather than confrontation.

There are other factors which have influenced the positive response to the program among Maine doctors. Hospital discharge data are public information. While the deliberations and conclusions of MMAP study groups are confidential, any person or organization with reasonable cause can get access to the computer files and carry out similar studies. A strong selling point of MMAP is that physicians will be in a much stronger position if they study, analyze, and act on the data before others do.

We have learned, however, that while practice variations can be leveled by feedback, where consensus regarding treatment does not exist, variations may recur in old areas or develop in new ones. As an example, disc surgery rates have begun to rise in new areas of Maine just as they have fallen in targeted areas. As effective as the feedback process is, lack of agreement regarding the indications for, and outcome of, disc surgery will continue to result in variations. We now believe that outcome studies are necessary, so that physicians have better information regarding indications for treatment, and both physicians and patients have more information on the risks and benefits of various medical interventions.

In 1983, when analysis of data showed increased mortality after prostatectomy, the urology study group undertook a patient-oriented, quality-of-life outcome study.[5] The majority of Maine's urologists voluntarily agreed to enroll their patients in this study. The study has now been completed, and publication is forthcoming. The study provides extensive data on the adverse effects of prostatectomy and will add significantly to our understanding of the risks and benefits of this frequently performed procedure. This information can be used to help both doctors and patients make more informed decisions regarding this type of surgery.

Following the lead of the urology study group's prostatectomy study, the orthopedic group is presently undertaking a prospective laminectomy outcome study to assess the indications for surgery versus conservative treatment in various patient groups. Similar projects by other study groups are also being planned.

ORGANIZING AN ASSESSMENT PROGRAM

Implementation of the small-area analysis concept within a state can occur in many ways. In Maine, physicians took the lead and have remained responsible for the program. We think this is ideal. But, obviously, the public availability of data opens the field to many organizations, such as hospitals, insurance carriers, business, labor, public interest groups, and government. The benefit of having doctors in the vanguard of analysis of this type seems obvious.

An assessment program can be structured in many forms, but support of organized medicine would appear essential. Endorsement by the state medical society gives immediate credibility; while lack of support--or worse, criticism--may be the kiss of death. A recognized, respected, and effective director can then develop the program. It seems particularly important in a program of this type that senior leadership be highly credible and acceptable to practicing doctors. Initially, the concept of the analysis of medical data and the study of practice variations can be very threatening to physicians. Effective leadership can overcome that problem. If such leadership is not present, however, the potential for rejection of the concept and failure of the program is very real. Funding also is essential. While physicians in Maine have worked largely on a voluntary basis, data analysis is expensive, and meeting and administrative costs must be met. The initial foundation funding of the Maine project is gradually being replaced by third-party insurance carriers.

168

As previously noted, we feel strongly that organization into specialty study groups has been much more effective than orientation to multi-specialty hospital or regional medical groups, though the latter might work well in other states. While reporting regularly to the director and the advisory committee, our study groups have been fairly autonomous. They have chosen their own fields of study and have developed individual, though similar, techniques of physician participation, education, and feedback.

IMPLICATIONS FOR MEDICAL CARE COSTS

Finally, a word about medical care costs. The emphasis of MMAP is on education and quality of care. It is clear, however, that when high rates of medical treatment are decreased, there is considerable cost savings. We can directly attribute a reduction of millions of dollars in health care costs to the work of MMAP. That achievement is, however, a by-product of our work. It is not its major focus. We are pleased that health care dollars have been conserved, but remain firmly committed to the notion that our program's success is based on the more fundamental goal of enhancing the quality of medical care, in this instance, through the analysis of physician practice patterns and outcome studies.

Figure 1. 1984 U.S. laminectomy rates, all pay sources in Maine, U.S., and census regions.

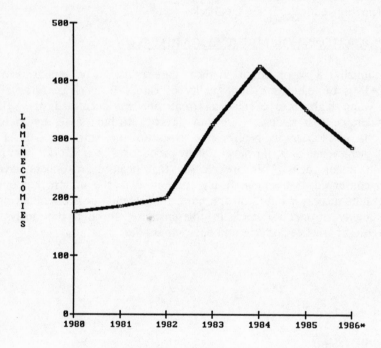

*1986 projected from Jan.-Sept.

Figure 2. Maine workers' compensation laminectomy trend extended to 1985-1986.

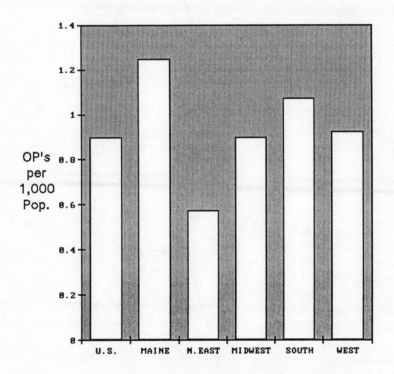

Any OP = ICD-9-CM Code 80.5-80.59

Figure 3. 1980-1986 workers' compensation laminectomies.

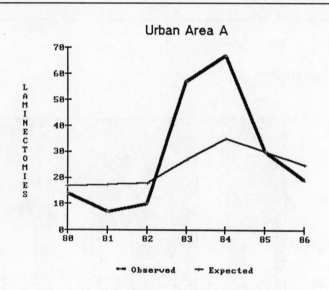

Urban Area A

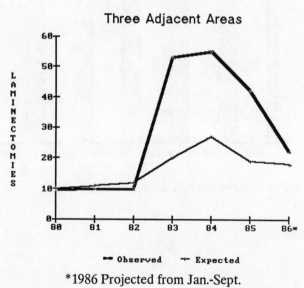

Three Adjacent Areas

*1986 Projected from Jan.-Sept.

Figure 4. Admissions for central Maine area children: four pediatric conditions.

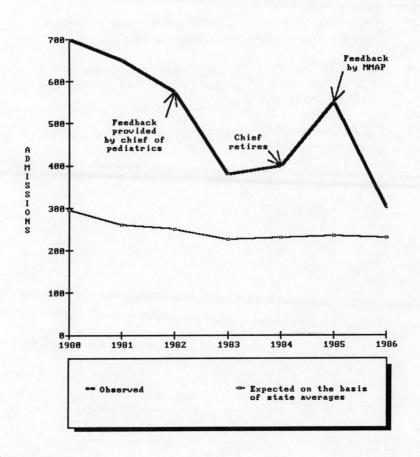

NOTES

1. J. Wennberg and A. Gittelsohn, "Small Area Variations in Health Care Delivery," *Science,* 183(1973): 1102-1108.

2. J. Wennberg, "Dealing with Medical Practice Variations: A Proposal for Action," *Health Affairs,* 3(1984): 26-33.

3. *Confronting Regional Variations--The Maine Approach,* (Chicago: American Medical Association, 1986).

4. R.K. Beals and N.W. Hickam, "Industrial Injuries of the Back and Extremities," *Journal of Bone and Joint Surgery,* 54A(1972): 1593-1611.

5. Publications forthcoming, Maine Medical Assessment Program, Augusta, Maine.

Chapter 9

Quality in the Prepaid Health Care Setting: The Federal Perspective*

Catherine F. Cleland, M.B.A.

Ever since the passage in 1973 of the Health Maintenance Organization Act (P.L.93-222), the federal government has had a keen interest in the quality of care provided to enrollees of prepaid health care plans. The focus of the government's interest has shifted over the years, however. The shift in focus reflects: 1) changes in the government's relationship to the prepaid health care industry; 2) the growth in the importance of quality as a policy issue; and 3) changes in the state-of-the-art of quality assurance and assessment.

From 1973 to the present, the federal government has maintained regulatory oversight of the HMO industry. This role, however, has always been combined with other significant functions. For instance, from 1973 to 1981, the government was the industry's chief financier, providing grants and loans to large numbers of developing prepaid plans. During this period, industry promotion was also an important federal function. Promotion was carried out through active market development initiatives such as business and community education programs and the recruitment of sponsors for start-up HMOs. Technical assistance was provided in areas of industry need such as planning, management information systems, and board development.[1-4]

---

*The views expressed in this chapter are those of the author and should not be construed as representing Health Care Financing Administration on Department of Health and Human Services policy.

When the HMO Medicare risk contract provisions of the Tax Equity and Fiscal Responsibility Act (TEFRA) were implemented formally in 1985 after more than two years of experience on a demonstration basis, the government assumed a major new role relative to HMOs as a purchaser of services for Medicare beneficiaries. In June 1987, this purchaser role took on an added dimension when the Health Care Financing Adminstration (HCFA) implemented the Health Maintenance Organization/Competitive Medical Plan* (HMO/CMP) external quality assessment program. At that time, Peer Review Organizations (PROs) had their mission expanded to include the assessment of the quality of care in HMOs and CMPs holding Medicare risk contracts. (See Chapter 5.)

The full impact of this expanded PRO mandate will become clear in the years ahead. For the present, however, it appears that 1987 will be seen as a watershed period for the HMO industry in that quality joined cost as a major policy issue. This outcome was the result of a convergence of forces from enrollees, employers, government, and the HMO industry itself. Under the Freedom of Information Act, the results of the PRO review of HMO/CMP quality will be available to the public. Thus, no longer will quality problems be dealt with quietly within the confines of a single organization or medical staff. Quality has effectively become a matter of public knowledge. The ripple effect of quality problems will be far reaching and will impact on market image. We will see, most likely, a heightened awareness of quality from the boards and senior managers of most HMOs and CMPs. This heightened awareness should have a pervasive influence on all aspects of HMO/CMP operations, including the allocation of resources.

---

*A competitive medical plan (CMP) is a prepaid, at-risk health care organization which meets the TEFRA requirements for eligibility to contract with HCFA on a risk basis. The requirements for CMP eligibility are more flexible than those for HMO qualification. For instance, CMPs may limit benefits, be experience rated, be a line of business of a state-licensed entity, and cover services provided out of plan.

Under the HMO/CMP external quality assessment program, strong incentives exist for individual HMO/CMPs to have rigorous internal quality assurance programs. Accordingly, we will undoubtedly see significant advances in the monitoring of the quality of care delivered in these plans. (See Chapter 10.) Innovations will come from HMO/CMPs motivated both to stay a step ahead of external review bodies and to use the available public information about quality as a marketing advantage over other prepaid and fee-for-service organizations. As a result of a congressional mandate in the Omnibus Budget Reconciliation Act of 1986, the Medicare program will be initiating quality review for ambulatory physician services covered by Medicare Part B. This review will not start until 1989, however, and then only on a "pilot study" basis. Thus, HMO/CMPs should be in the lead in furthering ambulatory quality monitoring techniques.

To fully appreciate the philosophy underlying the federal government's stance toward quality in HMO/CMPs, it is important to understand the context within which the government relates to HMO/CMPs in its various roles. The government's two current roles of regulator and purchaser provide a constructive tension with regard to quality that both balance and challenge each other's premises and strategies. In the regulatory role, the HMO/CMP's internal system for quality assurance is the principal focus of the government's attention. In the purchasing role, as will be discussed below, the focus is on the external assessment of the care actually delivered in the HMO/CMP. The interplay between these two foci of attention enhances the effectiveness and utility of each.

THE GOVERNMENT AS REGULATOR

In 1973, the federal government established statutory authority for oversight of the HMO industry in the quality assurance (QA) area. Congress saw HMOs as a promising alternative to fee-for-service medical care because they offered opportunities to provide comprehensive, coordinated health care at lower costs. However, since the cost reductions in HMOs were achieved through tight controls on the utilization of services, Congress wanted to be sure that the quality of health care in these organizations was not compromised. Thus, the first QA regulations for HMOs were published in 1974. They remain unchanged today.

Since HMOs are private entities, these regulations place the responsibility for quality assurance on each HMO. The HMO is to oversee the quality of its care by implementing systems to identify problems and take appropriate action to correct any deficiencies so identified. Underlying this approach is the assumption that a well-designed quality assurance program in an HMO will yield sufficient oversight of the plan's medical practice and administrative procedures such that any serious breaches of quality in the plan will be detected and readily corrected. This assumption was a long-standing one within the HMO industry, but it had not been empirically tested. The thrust of the government's regulatory focus thus has been to hold an HMO accountable for the functioning of its QA programs rather than to dictate either the parameters by which the actual quality of care within the organization should be judged or the standards to which it should conform.

Following the implementation of the 1974 regulations, the government-developed technical assistance materials to aid HMOs in establishing QA programs. In 1979, the "Quality Assurance Strategy for HMOs" was released by the Office of HMOs (OHMO) of the U.S. Public Health Service.[5] This document described the state-of-the-art standards of QA for HMOs at that time. Based on this document, standards for QA programs were later developed by the National Committee for Quality Assurance, an HMO-industry-sponsored organization.[6] In July 1986, OHMO circulated draft "QA Guidelines for HMOs and CMPs," which expanded on the earlier 1979 document and reflected the changes in the criteria of quality assurance in the intervening seven years.[7] This draft has gone through a number of revisions, the most recent being promulgated by HCFA's office of Prepaid Health Care in February 1988.[8] These drafts describe a model QA system for HMO/CMPs which is rigorous, comprehensive, and entails a much more aggressive approach to internal QA than ever before. As of this writing, the final guidelines are pending.

THE GOVERNMENT AS PURCHASER

When the federal government awarded the HMO/CMP risk contracts in April 1985, it added the role of purchaser of HMO/CMP services to its ongoing role of regulator.* By the late 1970s, the Reagan Administration and Congress had identified HMO/CMPs as vehicles for both reducing Medicare costs and lowering the government's profile with respect to benefit and payment decisions for Medicare beneficiaries.[9] Because HMO/CMPs are responsible for both providing health care to enrollees and financing those services, they have unique control over both the cost and quality of the benefits provided. Similarly, their products can be tailored to the local marketplace. Often an HMO/CMP package is attractive to the consumer because it offers a broad range of benefits for lower out-of-pocket costs and requires no claims forms. Efficient use of services by physicians is promoted through a combination of financial incentives and utilization controls.

It was this perspective that led to the government's being authorized by TEFRA to contract with HMO/CMPs to provide care to Medicare beneficiaries on a risk basis. Under the program, the government would pay the HMO/CMP a fixed monthly amount equal to 95 percent of what it would otherwise pay for the care of an average beneficiary of the same age and sex living in the same county. This amount is called the "adjusted average per capita cost" (AAPCC). Because of the economies HMOs had achieved for patients under age 65, it was widely believed that the Medicare benefit package could be provided by an HMO/CMP at considerably less than 95 percent of the fee-for-service average. The HMO/CMP would then be able to provide supplemental benefits to enrollees with these savings. However, should the HMO/CMP be unable to provide care within the financial limits imposed by the AAPCC, it would assume the loss. Under these arrangements, the government began to award demonstration contracts to HMO/CMPs to serve Medicare beneficiaries on a risk basis in 1982.

---

*Prior to this program, it was possible for a Medicare beneficiary to receive care in an HMO, but only on a cost-reimbursement basis. The option was not heavily utilized. The risk contract program brought the government into the role of purchaser in a major way.

Although the advantages of HMO/CMPs to Medicare enrollees appeared clear, the potential for HMO/CMPs to underserve enrollees and therein compromise the quality of care being delivered also existed. Congressional concern about this possibility led to two major pieces of legislation.

The Consolidated Omnibus Reconciliation Act (COBRA, P.L. 99-272) of 1985 amended the PRO statute and explicitly stated that PROs were required to conduct "peer review activities" on services provided by HMOs and CMPs holding Medicare risk contracts. (See Chapter 5.) This review was stipulated to begin in 1987. The specific services to be reviewed were not stipulated, however. Specificity was forthcoming in the Omnibus Budget Reconciliation Act (OBRA, P.L. 99-509) of October 1986. This legislation explicitly mandated that the review determine whether the *quality* of both inpatient *and* outpatient care in HMO/CMPs with Medicare risk contracts meets professionally recognized standards of health care, including whether appropriate health care services have not been provided or have been provided in inappropriate settings.

HCFA had been preparing for this legislation for some time. In fact, in early 1985, the Health Standards and Quality Bureau of HCFA, which manages the PRO program, had convened an Ad Hoc PRO/HMO Quality Review Committee. This committee was made up of representatives from the Group Health Association of America (GHAA), the American Medical Care and Review Association (AMCRA), and the American Medical Peer Review Association (AMPRA). The National Committee for Quality Assurance (NCQA) was given a contract to serve as staff to the committee. The charge to the Ad Hoc Committee was to develop a methodology for conducting inpatient and ambulatory review of HMOs and CMPs using existing data collection mechanisms for Medicare hospital discharges. NCQA submitted its final report in June 1985.[10]

The report recommended review of HMO/CMP cases which were admitted to a hospital for a selected number of conditions. These conditions were chosen because a hospital admission could represent substandard care at the ambulatory level. This approach to quality assessment owed much to the pioneering word of Drs. David Rutstein, Joyce Craddick, and Joseph Gonnella.[11-13] (See Chapters 2, 3, and 6.) It was to be incorporated, with a few modifications, into the final scope of work for the HMO/CMP external review methodology to be described later.[14,15]

This inpatient-triggered review of ambulatory care was to be the first government-sponsored review of the quality of care delivered in the privacy of physicians' offices. Thus, the new role of the government as purchaser of HMO/CMP care on a risk basis brought with it a commmitment to expanded review. An external review methodology would thus be developed and implemented to complement the government's preexisting and ongoing focus on internal HMO/CMP quality assurance programs. We shall now turn our attention to each of these approaches.

INTERNAL HMO/CMP QUALITY ASSURANCE PROGRAMS

As discussed earlier, HMO/CMPs are required by the original HMO Act of 1973 to have a quality assurance program which encompasses both inpatient and outpatient care. The "Quality Assurance Guidelines for HMOs and CMPs" were designed to provide guidance to HMO/CMPs regarding the government's expectations of their programs. HCFA intended the draft guidelines to be a launching pad for HMO/CMP internal QA efforts but did not want to stifle innovation by HMO/CMPs committed to intensive QA efforts, particularly in the ambulatory area. Thus, the guidelines are not viewed as rigid requirements, but rather as a description of the type of incisive QA program HMO/CMPs should develop. HMO/CMPs are encouraged to adopt alternative approaches with the proviso that they be equally rigorous and meet the regulations. The draft guidelines further reinforce the government's commitment to quality of care for Medicare beneficiaries enrolled in prepaid organizations.

The theme of the draft guidelines is that each HMO/CMP must take responsibility for having a rigorous quality assurance program. In order to do this, the board and senior management of the plan must make a realistic assessment of the areas in the organization where quality of care may be most vulnerable. (See Chapter 10.) Results of findings should be reported regularly to the board and senior management, and action should be taken when problems are found.

The Model HMO/CMP Quality Assurance Program Described in the "Guidelines"

The guidelines specify three factors as central to a successful HMO/CMP quality assurance program. They are: 1) the organization's structure and approach; 2) the structure of the QA system itself; and 3) the multi-dimensional scope of the QA program.

The organization's structures and approach

Each HMO/CMP should be structured in such a way that quality monitoring occurs at multiple levels within the organization. (See Chapter 10.) The board and senior management must be knowledgeable about areas of potential vulnerability within their organization, and their actions should be consistent with a sense of accountability for the quality of care delivered. A written QA plan with goals, objectives, and a timetable for implementation should serve as a blueprint for the QA system. The QA plan should address the role to be played by each part of the organization in the quality assurance effort.

Peer review is a fundamental part of any QA program, providing the medical expertise and credibility necessary for a meaningful program. The QA program should be managed by a physician, and a multispecialty team of physicians should work with him or her to implement it. When the activities of nonphysicians are being evaluated, appropriate representation from those professional groups should be included. All participating physicians and other health professionals should understand how their activities will be evaluated, how they can take an active role in the effort, and what to expect if problems are identified in their practices.

For the QA activities to be effective, there must be adequate program staff and data systems. QA can be very labor intensive, particularly when medical records of individuals are being evaluated at widely dispersed locations. (See Chapter 2.) The HMO/CMP must ensure that the reviewing staff is fully qualified and trained to use the criteria developed for the review. Final judgments of the quality of care delivered in individual cases should always be made by peers. Automated data systems which collect and report clinical data facilitate review activities and enhance the efficiency of the process. Throughout the review process, confidentiality of patient-specific information must be protected.

Though the implementation of the QA program will fall under the purview of a specific department, all employees of the HMO/CMP should be informed of the importance of QA to the organization. (See Chapter 10.) They might be aware of practices in the HMO/CMP which could affect negatively both the quality of the care being delivered and, actually, the perception of the quality of that care. If employees are alerted to the priority of improving quality, they will report incidents or situations they might otherwise ignore and thereby serve as a source of constructive suggestions to enhance quality. In addition, employees may enhance their own performance, particularly in relation to the enrollees, as a result of the HMO/CMP's "quality minded" approach permeating all activities.

A sensitive issue within some sectors of the HMO/CMP industry has been the delegation of QA responsibilities to either participating hospitals or medical groups with established QA programs of their own. In view of the HMO/CMP board's responsibilities for the quality of care provided in its organization, the judgment that must be made is which functions should be delegated and how intensive oversight should be in these situations. The possibilities range from conducting a full-scale QA program with no reliance on any external QA systems, to validating periodically a sample of the results of the delegated QA activities as a supplement to interim reports, to simply reviewing such reports with no further verification.

In deciding which approach to adopt, the HMO/CMP should consider three factors. First, how are payments to the providers structured, and do they create incentives to underserve enrollees? Second, what percentage of the provider's revenues are dependent upon the HMO/CMP? Third, what is the scope and track record of the quality assurance program? For instance, if the HMO/CMP pays for services in such a way that places a level of financial risk on an individual provider (i.e., physician, medical group, or hospital), which could be an incentive to underserve enrollees, then delegating review may be ill-advised. On the other hand, the need for a supplementary QA structure is greatly reduced if the provider serves the HMO almost exclusively (i.e., almost all of its revenues come from the HMO/CMP) or where the identities of the HMO/CMP and the provider are otherwise closely interrelated. In the latter case, however, the board of the HMO/CMP must still approve the provider's QA program, establish a monitoring plan to assure that the program continues to meet its expectations, and receive regular reports on the results of the review. If problems are found and the provider does not take appropriate corrective action, then the HMO/CMP must act. The important point is that the HMO/CMP board must know what is happening to its enrollees and have an agreed-upon approach to take action to address problems as they arise.

The structure of the HMO/CMP QA system

The structure of the QA system should combine the classic "QA feedback loop" with a technique to identify problems in areas of known vulnerability.[16] Problem identification should be the driving force behind the entire QA system. The problems selected for examination should be important to the health of the enrolled population; otherwise, the QA effort will be hollow. The QA feedback loop is a well-known method for ensuring that once problems are documented, recommendations for action will be formulated, implemented and then re-evaluated to ensure that change has occurred.[17]

The HMO/CMP can identify its areas of vulnerability in two ways. First, there are a number of conditions or procedures which carry with them a high risk for possibly adverse outcomes. Similarly, there generally are a number of high-volume or high-risk conditions or procedures in each plan. These conditions and procedures exist for virtually all clinical specialties and services, regardless of the patient's payment arrangements. A group of medical professionals for each specialty should be assembled to identify these potential areas of vulnerability. Using the Delphi method or Nominal Group Technique, the group can develop a consensus on a set of indicators that should be monitored on an ongoing basis to determine whether the process and outcomes of care are acceptable in these areas of potential vulnerability.

Second, there are areas of vulnerability for HMO/CMPs which arise from their unique administrative and financial attributes. Specifically, although the financial risk and incentives found in most HMO/CMPs are intended to motivate physicians to prescribe services efficiently, they lend themselves to the possibility of physicians underusing, delaying, or even denying needed services. Other administrative features of HMO/CMPs, such as tight utilization controls (which may lead to premature discharges, delayed access, and so on); use of only participating specialists (which may create an accessibility issue); or the requirements for coordinated care (which may necessitate time-consuming prior authorization) can also impinge on the quality of care provided. (See Chapter 1.) Each of these features differentiate the HMO/CMP environment from the fee-for-service sector and should be closely scrutinized to ensure that enrollees are not placed at risk.

By relying on specific, predefined indicators of quality, the quality assessment process can be focused and efficient (see note 17). Once the indicators are selected by physicians and other health professionals, screens can be applied to data normally found in the claims payment system or in any system that uses encounter forms to track utilization. These screens trigger review of any case in which one of the indicators is present. (See Chapters 2 and 6.) The indicators selected for use as screens should be oriented to the processes and outcomes of care. Indicators that can be monitored include, for example, avoidable acute inpatient admissions (discussed later in the external review section of this chapter), low-birth-weight babies, abnormal Pap smears, two visits in the same week for the same problem, drug reactions, unplanned returns to the operating room, and so on.[18] When a case falls outside the specified parameters, it can be referred to the appropriate health care professionals to determine whether questions of quality exist. Criteria developed by physicians and other health professionals are used to identify situations where in-depth review of the medical record is necessary. If substandard quality of care is found, action can be taken with respect to the professionals involved.

As data are collected on each of the important indices of care, patterns and trends can be observed that will reveal incidence norms for the enrolled population and participating providers. Questionable patterns or trends can be pursued using the QA loop methodology alluded to above (see note 17).

The multidimensional scope of the QA program

The quality assurance program should be multidimensional; that is, it should address all the types of care provided, or arranged for, by the HMO/CMP, as well as the full range of quality issues that can arise in a prepaid setting. To be credible, the QA program for a comprehensive health service delivery system must itself be comprehensive in addressing all settings of care, departments, medical disciplines, and enrolled populations. Furthermore, all the different attributes of quality--availability, accessibility, acceptability, continuity, and so on--as well as technical quality must be examined. (See Chapters 1 and 2.) Since quality problems can exist anywhere in this spectrum, the HMO/CMP should have an ongoing surveillance system to detect practices or situations that warrant further evaluation. As stated above, the various departments and disciplines should work with the QA committee to select a priority listing of quality indicators in their area. Several of these should be tracked simultaneously at all times. Groups of indicators can be rotated for broadest surveillance. These indicators should be followed over time with routine feedback on individual and collective performance.

Examples of areas that an HMO should monitor include the following:

- Appropriateness of the diagnosis and treatment (technical quality);
- Appropriateness of the level of care at which the patient is receiving treatment (accessibility and technical quality);
- Availability of medically necessary emergency services 24 hours a day, seven days a week (availability and accessibility);
- Locations of providers in relation to enrolled population (accessibility);
- Ratio of full-time-equivalent primary and specialty providers to the enrolled population (accessibility);
- Waiting times in the office and for appointments (accessibility);
- Disenrollment rates (acceptability);
- Frequency of visits for chronic conditions or well-baby care (continuity); and
- Timely referrals to appropriate specialists (accessibility). (See notes 6, 19, and 20.)

There are also a number of other sources of information which the HMO/CMP can use to track the performance of its delivery system. Enrollee and staff surveys can provide critical data on the day-to-day operation of the plan. These data can be particularly useful in assessing availability and accessibility of care. An evaluation of complaints and grievances can reveal clusters of problems in addition to highlighting individual incidents. Analysis of utilization data can help pinpoint issues of quality where continuity of care is a concern and where high-cost cases may be indicative of inappropriate treatment plans.

A QA program monitoring the various indicators will yield important data which the board and management can use to determine problem areas within their delivery system. There are two remaining factors, however, which greatly influence the quality of care provided in the HMO/CMP and the ability of the board, management and QA committee to perform proper oversight.

First, the physicians and other health professionals must be qualified to perform their services, and the facilities must be safe and well equipped. (See Chapter 1.) Without these prerequisites, quality of care will be difficult to achieve even with the best QA program. Therefore, rigorous screening of all providers should be conducted. Information on physicians--such as the number of malpractice actions brought against them, revocation or suspension of a license, investigation by the Drug Enforcement Administration/Bureau of Narcotics and Dangerous Drugs, criminal convictions, curtailment or suspension of medical privileges, or censure by a state or county medical society--should be obtained and reviewed systematically by the HMO/CMP before contracts are signed. Prior to each contract renewal, updated information on each of the above parameters, along with data compiled on each physician's performance, should be presented to the board committee which oversees provider relations.

The importance for health care organizations of the credentialing of health professionals has been underscored by the passage of the Health Care Quality Improvement Act of 1986 (P.L.99-660) (See note 8). This law, which is still awaiting an appropriation, establishes a national data bank on physicians and other health care professionals who have been subject to malpractice payments, disciplined by an appropriate body, or had clinical privileges at a health care institution adversely affected for more than 30 days. Under the law, hospitals and HMOs will be required to report actions of their peer review committees to the State Board of Medical Examiners, which will then transmit the information to the national data bank. Hospitals must request information from the national data bank when a physician or other health care professional applies for staff privileges and once every two years thereafter. HMOs may, but are not required to, access the information. The law also provides immunity against liability for damages to members of bodies which conduct professional review activities or to persons providing information to such bodies.

The second factor that affects an HMO/CMP's ability to perform QA activities is the adequacy and legibility of documentation in the medical record. Not only must the HMO/CMP be able to ascertain what care was provided and when, but the physician also must be able to reference the history and physical examinations, treatment plans, consultations, medications, allergies, and other information to ensure the appropriateness of care. An HMO/CMP's interest in promoting good recordkeeping is twofold: the organization will be able to verify what transpired in the course of treatment and to respond to the needs of external review organizations, thereby avoiding the possible imposition of harsh penalties, as will be discussed below (see note 8).

EXTERNAL REVIEW OF THE QUALITY OF CARE IN HMO/CMP RISK CONTRACTORS

Quality Safeguards

In creating the HMO/CMP option for Medicare beneficiaries, Congress and the Reagan Administration proceeded with care. Lessons had been learned from previous capitation programs in California, and safeguards were built into the design of this new Medicare benefit.[21] From early on, the PROs were slated to conduct external quality review of HMO/CMP Medicare services. Also included in the various statutes were other controls intended to enhance quality. For instance, HMO/CMPs are prohibited from having Medicare or Medicaid beneficiaries constitute more than 50 percent of their enrollment. The rationale for this limitation is that, to be acceptable to the Medicare program, an HMO/CMP has to be sufficiently competitive in the commercial marketplace to attract at least 50 percent of its enrollees from private employers. The standard of quality necessary to attract and retain the commercial population should imply an acceptable level of quality for Medicare and Medicaid enrollees.

Another safeguard is that Medicare enrollees can disenroll from an HMO/CMP at any time. The disenrollment becomes effective at the beginning of the next month. Thus, if Medicare beneficiaries do not find HMO/CMP care to their liking, they are free to switch out of the HMO/CMP at any time. This provision ensures continuing freedom of choice for the beneficiary between care in the fee-for-service sector and in an HMO/CMP. Finally, Medicare risk contracts may be awarded only to qualified HMOs and eligible CMPs. For an HMO to be judged qualified by the federal government and a CMP to be deemed eligible, it must, among many other requirements, provide comprehensive health care services and have an acceptable quality assurance program.

Conventional wisdom would suggest that these requirements should protect beneficiaries from substandard care quite well. However, these requirements are lacking what purchasers desire most in the realm of quality--proof of its level. Major advances have been made in our ability to objectively assess quality. (See Chapter 2.) Congressional action in 1985 and 1986 clearly indicated that it wanted these measures to be applied to both the inpatient and outpatient care being provided to Medicare beneficiaries in HMO/CMPs.

The External Review Methodology

The review of HMO/CMP risk contractors began on June 1, 1987. The review is being performed by 27 PROs and one Quality Review Organization (QRO).* The methodology for the review represents a unique and progressive approach to quality assessment. It is efficient, focused and, above all, its intensity is a function of the effectiveness of the HMO's own QA program. The objectives

---

*A Quality Review Organization (QRO) is an organization that meets the requirements of a PRO, but performs quality review only of HMO services in a given state(s). The Omnibus Budget Reconciliation Act of 1986 allowed organizations other than the designated PRO from each state with an HMO Medicare risk contract to compete to perform review of the care provided under the contract. This competition was permitted in up to 25 states. One QRO, Quality Quest, Inc., of Excelsior, MN, initially a joint venture between InterStudy, Inc., and the Minnesota PRO, was awarded contracts to conduct the HMO/CMP review in Illinois, Kansas, and Missouri. With two exceptions, for the remaining states in which there is an HMO/CMP with a Medicare risk contract, the review is performed by the PRO of that state. The exceptions are Arizona and Hawaii, whose HMO/CMP review is performed by the California PRO. In the remainder of this chapter, the discussion of PRO review also applies to QRO review.

of the system are: to provide strong incentives for an HMO/CMP to have a rigorous, comprehensive internal QA program; to identify HMO/CMPs which may be providing substandard quality of care to Medicare beneficiaries; and to give HMO/CMPs an opportunity to correct deficiencies identified by external reviewers.

PRO/QROs are assigned seven tasks which will enable them to accomplish these objectives (see note 15). They are:

- Reviewing the performance of the HMO/CMP's internal QA program;
- Conducting individual record review for selected types of care;
- Compiling profiles of HMO/CMP care;
- Performing community outreach to educate Medicare beneficiaries about their rights under the HMO/CMP option and reviewing complaints about HMO/CMP care;
- Overseeing HMO/CMP corrective action plans;
- Initiating recommendations for civil monetary penalties; and
- Initiating recommendations for sanctions.

The "three-level" system of review

The first two tasks mentioned above serve as the foundation for the "three-level" system of review: namely, limited, basic, and intensified. Initially, an HMO/CMP is assigned to limited or basic review depending upon an assessment by the PRO/QRO of the strength of its internal QA program. (See Figure 1.) Movement from the initially assigned level to intensified review would occur if the PRO/QRO's review process uncovers deficiencies in the HMO/CMP's own review process that exceed a specified threshold (to be discussed later). Once under intensified review, an HMO/CMP can move back to limited or basic review if the number of deficiencies found by the PRO remains below the threshold for a specified period of time. A reassignment of an HMO/CMP from basic to limited review requires a reassessment of the strength of its QA program. The HMO/CMP must request this reassessment.

The concept of limited review is that the HMO/CMP's own QA system is substituting for a portion of the PRO's review. For this reason, to qualify for limited review, the HMO/CMP must have a QA system which mirrors the type of review to be performed by

190

the PRO. Thus, the HMO/CMP must demonstrate that its program incorporates such features as: review of individual cases of patient care; use of reasonable sampling methods to select cases; coverage of all settings; attention to quality, appropriateness, and access problems; and corrective action for substandard care. To determine the appropriateness of the "limited" review designation, the PRO also reviews a sample of cases previously reviewed by the HMO/CMP to evaluate the validity of the original review. If the PRO finds deficiencies in 5 percent of the cases so evaluated, or a minimum of six cases, whichever is higher, the HMO/CMP is subject to basic review even if its QA program has met all the other criteria.

Once the HMO/CMP is assigned to the limited or basic level, review is organized around the five categories of cases given below. In the review of these cases, such criteria as technical quality of care, timeliness, appropriateness of the setting, and timing of discharge can be addressed depending on their relevance to the particular category. The volume of cases reviewed will be greater for basic review than for limited review. The number of cases for intensified review is even greater. The five categories are:

- Inpatient admissions for 13 conditions which may be associated with substandard ambulatory care;
- A random sample of inpatient cases;
- Non-trauma deaths in all settings;
- Transfers from nonparticipating hospitals to participating hospitals; and
- Hospital readmissions within 30 days of discharge.

There will also be focused review of ambulatory care for conditions which rarely result in hospitalization.

In addition, as part of limited review, the PRO will have to regularly validate the HMO/CMP's internal QA program through an ongoing review of a subsample of cases previously evaluated by the HMO/CMP. The size of this sample to be reviewed is a function of the number of Medicare beneficiaries enrolled in the plan. Table 1 shows the five categories of cases to be reviewed and the size of the sample to be selected for each level of review.

An HMO/CMP will continue under its assigned level of review unless the PRO finds deficiencies in 5 percent of, or a minimum of six, cases (whichever is higher) which were not identified by the

HMO/CMP or, if identified, were not acted upon. Should this happen, a higher level of review is triggered. As can be seen in Table 1, intensified review involves a significantly higher volume of review than limited or basic review. It is expected that intensified review will be sufficiently onerous for an HMO/CMP that it will act to improve its internal QA program immediately. If, after six months at the intensified level, the number of deficiencies identified falls below the 5 percent or six case threshold, then the HMO/CMP will return to basic review. The HMO/CMP can also request limited review at this time. If requested, the PRO/QRO would reassess the HMO/CMP's internal QA system to ensure that the problems originally triggering the basic level have been corrected.

Conducting individual case review for the five categories of cases

In addition to the incentives for HMO/CMPs to have effective QA programs, the other distinctive feature of the external HMO/CMP review methodology is the examination of the linkage between an HMO/CMP inpatient admission and the quality of care provided to the case in the ambulatory setting.

The external review methodology requires PRO/QRO to review the quality of HMO/CMP ambulatory care received by beneficiaries being hospitalized for any one of 13 different conditions:

- Diabetic complications;
- Acute appendicitis;
- Hypertensive problems;
- Gastrointestinal catastrophes;
- Gangrene of an extremity;
- Operations for breast malignancy;
- Malignant neoplasm of genito-urinary organs;
- Adverse drug reactions;
- Cellulitis;
- Malignant neoplasm of colon;
- Hypokalemia;
- Septicemia; and
- Pulmonary embolism (see note 15).

The ability of PROs to efficiently identify cases in any of these conditions is made possible by the fact that hospitals must submit to HCFA a standard claim form, the "UB-82," for all their Medicare discharges. HMO/CMP patients are identified as such on the UB-82. The HCFA fiscal intermediary notifies the PRO of any cases hospitalized with these 13 conditions, the PRO in turn notifies the HMO/CMP of these cases and asks it to submit the relevant ambulatory records for review.

For three of the four remaining categories of cases to be reviewed, namely the random sample of inpatient cases, hospital transfers within 30 days, and hospital readmissions, generic screens must be used. These categories of cases are identical to those being reviewed by the PROs under PPS and the same generic screens are used. (See Chapters 5 and 6.) Inpatient care associated with the 13 conditions will also be reviewed as will the outpatient care between hospital admissions for the readmission cases.

The fifth category of cases included in the PRO scope of work is non-trauma deaths of HMO/CMP Medicare beneficiaries in any setting. Review of a random sample of such deaths will determine whether the death resulted from substandard, inappropriate, or delayed care.

Compilation and analysis of profiles

The findings of the external review are profiled by the PRO on an HMO/CMP-specific and physician-specific basis. Profiles are a useful tool to determine whether the deficiencies found are due to overall poor performance on a particular type of case or to a particular physician. The review system is flexible in that if it appears the deficiencies which triggered intensified review are clustered in a few conditions or with a few physicians, the intensification will apply only to those conditions or physicians.

Profiles are also useful in evaluating the performance of physicians practicing with more than one HMO/CMP. The PRO/QRO will be able to merge the review results from all the HMO/CMPs with Medicare risk contracts in each state. If one physician has a low volume of Medicare cases in several HMO/CMPs, the magnitude of a problem with his or her practice may not be apparent by looking only at each HMO/CMP in isolation. Combining the review results will afford the PRO a unique perspective on a physician's entire Medicare HMO practice.

Community outreach

The purposes of the community outreach portion of PRO review are: to inform Medicare beneficiaries of the types of activities performed by the PRO; to educate beneficiaries about their rights; and to receive complaints from beneficiaries regarding the quality, accessibility, and adequacy of HMO/CMP care. Beneficiary complaints about quality must be investigated by the PRO through a review of the beneficiary's medical record. The PRO's findings are then reported back to the beneficiary. As with other types of review, if deficiencies exceed the 5 percent or six case threshold (whichever is higher), the intensity of the review will be increased.

Oversight for HMO/CMP corrective actions plans

As deficiencies are found, the PRO will inform the HMO/CMP of its findings and will allow a designated timeframe for the HMO/CMP to provide supplementary information. If the PRO is not convinced by the additional information that deficiencies did not indeed occur, it will ask the HMO/CMP for a corrective action plan to address the deficiencies noted. Monitoring will take place to assure that the plan is followed. Ongoing PRO review activities will continue as well. Oversight of corrective actions will cease when it becomes clear that the problems have been dealt with effectively. If progress is not made within a reasonable period of time, the PRO can impose harsher penalties, from recommending that the Medicare contract be terminated to recommending sanctions by the Office of the Inspector General of the Department of Health and Human Services. (See Chapter 6 for a discussion of similar issues with respect to hospital care under PPS.)

Recommendations to impose civil monetary penalties

Where a PRO finds that an HMO/CMP has failed to provide medically necessary services and that this failure has had an adverse impact on the patients affected, a penalty of $10,000 can be imposed on the HMO/CMP for each violation. Recommendations are made by the PRO to the Office of the Inspector General which makes the final determination. (See Chapter 6.)

Recommendations for sanctions

Gross and flagrant violations of professionally recognized standards of care must be reported to the Inspector General. Should the Inspector General uphold the PRO's finding, a financial penalty or expulsion from Medicare will result. The HMO/CMP as well as the physicians and/or hospitals involved can be subject to sanctions.

CONCLUSION

The external quality review methodology described above encourages HMO/CMPs to act to improve their own QA program. A combination of monitoring calibrated to the strengths of each HMO/CMP and a broad scope for the review should enable the PRO to efficiently focus its resources in HMO/CMP review, quickly detecting and addressing problem areas across the outpatient-inpatient spectrum, with minimal intrusion where good performance is documented.

A watershed period for HMO/CMPs has arrived with respect to quality. The cumulative effects of Congressional mandates for oversight of the quality of HMO/CMP care provided to Medicare beneficiaries, increased emphasis on quality by regulators and commercial purchasers, heightened awareness of quality by the public, and intensified pressures on the HMO industry to present an attractive alternative to fee-for-service have brought the industry to its current state of involvement with quality as a managerial, policy, and marketing issue. Together, these forces are powerful motivators for voluntary enhancement of quality assurance efforts by HMO/CMPs. The federal PRO external review effort not only will enable PRO/QROs to collect and report data on individual HMO/CMPs, but should also lead to the ability to compare these data across HMO/CMPs. This ability will further stimulate HMO/CMP QA efforts.

From the government's perspective, its regulator and purchaser roles have merged in such a way that not only requires HMO/CMPs to meet its requirements in the area of quality assessment, but also encourages them to go further. The internal and external quality review approaches are overlapping, mutually reinforcing, and ensure that senior HMO/CMP management will give greater recognition to the importance of QA. It should soon be clear to HMO/CMP board members and managers that the rigorous assurance of the quality of the care their HMO/CMP delivers, is, in the last analysis, in their plan's own best interest.   By assuring, measuring, and marketing good quality, HMO/CMP managers effectively can differentiate their plan in a very competitive environment.

Table 1

Five Categories of HMO/CMP Cases for PRO/QRO Review by the Sample Size for Three Different Levels of Review

Category of Cases   The Three Levels of Review and Sample Size

	Limited Review	Basic Review	Intensified Review
The 13 Conditions	50% of four conditions	50%	100%
Deaths (Non-trauma)	5%	10%	100%
Transfers	100%	100%	100%
Readmissions			
Within 7 Days	25%	50%	100%
Within 8-15 Days	25%	50%	100%
Within 16-30 Days	15%	25%	100%
Random Sample of Inpatient Cases	3%	3%	6%

Source: Adapted from Health Standards and Quality Bureau, Health Care Financing Administration, U.S. Department of Health and Human Services, "Scope of Work for PRO/QRO Review of HMO/CMO Medicare Risk Contractors," Washington, DC, March 1987.

Figure 1. The "three levels" of PRO/QRO review of HMOs/CMPs.

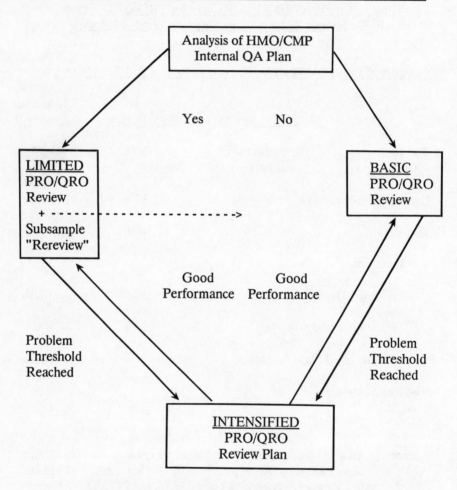

Source: Adapted from Health Standards and Quality Bureau, Health Care Financing Administration, U.S. Department of Health and Human Services, "Scope of Work for PRO/QRO Review of HMO/CMP Medicare Risk Contractors," Washington, DC, March 1987.

NOTES

1. Office of Health Maintenance Organizations, *A Guide to Development of Health Maintenance Organizations* (Washington, DC: Department of Health and Human Services, 1982).

2. Office of Health Maintenance Organizations, *HMO Critical Performance Measures* (Rockville, MD: Department of Health and Human Services, Spring 1983).

3. Office of Health Maintenance Organizations, *The Design, Selection and Implementation of a Management Information System for Health Maintenance Organizations* (vol. 1, revised) (Rockville, MD: Department of Health and Human Services, 1983).

4. Office of Health Maintenance Organizations, *HMO Governing Board Handbook* (Rockville, MD: Department of Health and Human Services, 1981).

5. Office of Health Maintenance Organizations, *Quality Assurance Strategy for HMOs* (Washington, DC: Department of Health and Human Services, 1979).

6. *Standards for the Evaluation of the Quality Assurance Program* (Washington, DC: National Committee for Quality Assurance, 1986).

7. Office of Prepaid Health Care, *Quality Assurance Guidelines for Health Maintenance Organizations and Competitive Medical Plans* (draft) (Washington, DC: Department of Health and Human Services, 1986).

8. Office of Prepaid Health Care, *Quality Assurance Guidelines for Health Maintenance Organizations and Competitive Medical Plans* (draft) (Washington, DC: Department of Health and Human Services, February 1988).

9. P.B. Ginsburg and G.M. Hackbarth, "Alternative Delivery Systems and Medicare," *Health Affairs,* 5(1986): 6-22.

10. *Recommendations of the Ad Hoc PRO/HMO Quality Review Committee to the Health Standards and Quality Bureau* (Baltimore, MD: National Committee for Quality Assurance, 1985).

11. D.D. Rutstein, et al., "Measuring the Quality of Medical Care, A Clinical Method," *New England Journal of Medicine,* 294(1976): 582-588.

12. J.S. Gonnella, D.Z. Louis, and J.J. McCord, "The Staging Concept --An Approach to the Assessment of Outcome and Ambulatory Care," *Medical Care,* 14(1976): 13-21.

13. J.W. Craddick and B.S. Bader, *Medical Management Analysis: A Systematic Approach to Quality Assurance and Risk Management: Volume 1, An Introduction* (Auburn, CA: Joyce W. Craddick, 1983).

14. L.I. Solberg, et al., *The Minnesota Project: An Innovative Approach to Ambulatory Care Quality Assurance* (unpublished report, February 1987).

15. Health Standards and Quality Bureau, *Scope of Work for PRO/QRO Review of HMO/CMP Medicare Risk Contractors* (Washington, DC: Department of Health and Human Services, 1987).

16. Health Standards and Quality Bureau, Health Care Financing Administration, *Handbook for the Conduct of Medical Care Evaluation Studies* (Washington, DC: Government Printing Office, 1978).

17. R.H. Palmer and H.R. Nesson, "A Review of Methods for Ambulatory Care Evaluations," *Medical Care,* 20(August 1982): 8.

18. S. Leary, "Building Blocks of an Effective QA Program," paper delivered at conference, Assuring Quality of Care in HMOs, Group Health Association of America, Phoenix, AZ, October 23-25, 1986.

19. *Accreditation Handbook of Ambulatory Health Care,* 1985-1986 ed. (Skokie, IL: Accreditation Association for Ambulatory Health Care, 1985).

20. *Ambulatory Health Care Standards Manual* (Chicago, IL: Joint Commission on Accreditation of Healthcare Organizations, 1986).

21. *A Report of the Prepaid Health Research, Evaluation, and Demonstration Project* (San Francisco, CA: California State Department of Health Service, 1981).

22. J.P. Weiner, "Assuring Quality of Care in HMOs: Past Lessons, Present Challenges, and Future Decisions," *GHAA Journal,* 7(1986): 10-27.

Chapter 10

Quality Assurance and Measurement Principles: The Perspective From One Health Maintenance Organization

Donald M. Berwick, M.D.

A story is told in quality control circles in industry. I cannot vouch for its accuracy, but it makes its point well. The story alleges that the American Congress and the Japanese Diet passed legislation at about the same time requiring more stringent emission standards for automobiles in their respective countries. In the United States, so goes the tale, the automobile industry almost immediately began holding national meetings to plan ways to get the legislation changed. In Japan, the automobile industry also began holding national meetings, but they were trying to plan the most efficient ways to produce better emission control systems.

Health care faces some choices, too. Today, we find enormous and increasing pressures to contain our costs, and somewhat newer but also increasing pressures to measure, control, and display our quality. How will we respond? Will we try to get the rules changed? Will we try mainly to justify our current practices and resist the onslaught of new regulations and tougher scrutiny? Or, will we take a leaf from Japan's lesson in the preceding story and search for better ways to deliver the best possible health care in these new times?

In this chapter, I will try to explore some principles which could guide a constructive response to the demand for the measurement and control of quality in American health care, partly by drawing lessons from one recent experiment in quality control at the Harvard Community Health Plan (HCHP), the largest staff-model health maintenance organization (HMO) in New England. But first, it may be helpful to review the pressures to which we all must respond today regarding quality. Why has quality control suddenly risen to the top rank in the national health care debate?

WHY QUALITY NOW?

The current surge of interest in quality derives its energy primarily, of course, from pressures on health care costs. Regulation, competition, prospective payment, and risk contracts are pressing health care producers of all types to try to hold their costs and prices down, and we may well be nearing the limits of our ability to contain at least some costs without placing patients at significant hazard. Without tools for measuring quality, we may never know when we cross that line.

But there are also other sources for today's concern about quality. We have, for example, strong evidence that physicians vary greatly among themselves in the rates at which they use health care resources. Over a decade ago, Professor John Wennberg and his colleagues compared the rates of surgical procedures in New England with those in Southern Norway and the West Midland region of England.[1] They found wide differences; gall bladder operations, for example, were nearly four times as common per inhabitant of New England as in the West Midlands. Hysterectomies and tonsillectomies were nearly five times as common in New England as in Norway. Subsequent research has shown that equally large differences exist among regions within the United States,[2] and even among doctors practicing in the same hospitals or medical groups.[3]

A rational public is unwilling to believe that patients subjected to that kind of variability in care are all receiving care of equal quality. Without measurement systems for quality, however, it is difficult to define correct practice patterns, and, worse, it is maliciously tempting to conclude (in the service of cost containment) that low utilization rates are best.

A third factor in the new demand for quality measurement is the increasing dominance in the medical marketplace of the purchaser, often in the guise of health benefits officers in corporations which choose among care systems for their employees. We are in transition today from a professionally dominated medical care system, in which the physician makes most of the relevant consumption choices, to a purchaser dominated system. With the profession in control, explicit information systems on quality are not usually required; professionals reign through trust and the sole authority to judge their own quality implicitly. In a purchaser dominated system, however, information on quality must be available for the purchaser to make informed choices. Today's health care consumers need to know about the quality of care they purchase, and they have the power to demand that information.

Fourth, we see today in health care a segmented market, with more types of demand than in the days when a more unified profession defined high-quality care. The HMO in which I work has both busy lawyers and isolated, poor, single parents among its members. "High-quality health care" has very different meanings for those two constituencies. The lawyer may need the quickest possible visit over a lunch hour, caring less about a close relationship with a physician, perhaps, than that care be competent, prompt, and take as little time as possible. The single mother from the inner city may desparately need continuity in her health care, long sessions addressing multiple health-related problems, and the freedom to be late for an appointment or to walk in unexpectedly. If such disparate clients are to choose correctly from among the health care options available to them, they must have information on the characteristics each of them regard as "quality" when they make their choices.

Increasing malpractice liability is a fifth force driving quality up on our agenda. It is common now to hope that, if we could control and measure quality, we might establish at least one line of defense against the rapidly rising costs of litigation in health care.

These forces--cost containment, variation in practice, purchaser needs, market segmentation, malpractice liability--compose a litany of "negative" pressures toward quality control; they urge quality control as a defensive strategy. "Positive" forces also exist which push us toward quality improvement as a new opportunity in health care, one which we might happily pursue even if the negative pressures were not upon us.

Think, for example, of the relatively new potential of information systems in health care today. New uses of computers in medicine, such as the automated medical record in the HCHP, or sophisticated new claims systems just starting to emerge, allow us now to aggregate data on health care patterns at a very high level, and thereby to search for forms of deficiency and excellence in health care that we could not easily find at lower levels of aggregation. We can now begin to find patterns of events too infrequent or subtle to notice in small, disaggregated data sets.

The potential of managed care, itself, offers further opportunities. Managed systems can introduce some hazards by putting increased pressure on costs, but they also create the capacity to respond to quality problems with a precision and scope not possible in a cottage industry. "Managed care" systems are only now really starting to manage care (in addition to managing costs), and their potential to improve care through thoughtful new methods of organization and management may be enormous. To do so, however, they will need tools through which to measure and control their care--tools for quality measurement.

THE STATE OF THE MEASUREMENT ART

Compared to these pressures demanding quality measurement, we have an embarrassing dearth of technologies to perform that measurement. In fact, though we have crossed the half-trillion dollar mark in health care in America, we still almost completely lack an applied technology to assess the quality of our industry.

By an applied technology for measurement, I mean one that is useful to decision makers in health care. Such a technology would have to have several features to be useful: First, it would have to produce timely information; that is, information yielded at a pace consistent with the metabolic rate of the health care manager. In organizations and departments, for example, health care managers make their decisions over weeks, or maybe months. The research literature on health care quality assessment tends, instead, to describe methods which yield information over years--much too slowly for the impatient, environmentally driven decision makers in today's health care systems.

Second, an applied technology for measurement would have to aggregate information at a level which matches the domain of choice for the decision maker. Chiefs of internal medicine need information about their department, not about the state of Maryland or the condition of American health care. Tools for managers must allow measurement within specific fields, and the research literature on quality assurance in health care does not yet offer such a focused technology.

Third, useful measurement technologies in health care must not be too costly. We have very little information on what is "too costly," but the HCHP, which today invests about one-third of 1 percent of its premium revenues in quality measurement, seems to be far ahead of most of the industry in its willingness to invest in the measurement process. The research models for measurement tend to be far too costly for general, regular use in today's medical marketplace.

A fourth feature of an applied technology, one entirely under-estimated in importance in the general literature on quality assurance, is the means to display findings efficiently for consumers of infor-mation. Among the great breakthroughs in industrial quality control was the development of visually effective charts and graphic devices through which managers could trace the quality of their production systems. Few managers of today's health care systems seem ac-quainted with even the seminal work of such researchers as Beverley Payne,[4] Robert Brook,[5] and John Williamson[6]--pioneers in health care quality assurance whose technical advances seem to remain inaccessible to day-to-day managers, in part perhaps because their findings and methods seem arcane and too complex for the rapid-fire needs of line management. To control quality, health care will need not just measurement tools, but also ways to display results that are as conventional, accessible, and easily understood as those used in financial accounting.

Finally, if health care quality measurement is to become an applied technology, it will have to deal with quality as a multidimen-sional concept. Too much of the research literature assumes that high quality is equivalent to the production of good health status outcomes. Oversimplified, this view of quality becomes flat and, since very little is known about the efficacy of many health care practices, sometimes paralytic. A richer view of quality recognizes: 1) in health care as in most enterprises, no one is good at everything, and few are poor at everything; and 2) a sensible definition of quality has many independent dimensions. As we shall see below, the measurement system being put into place at HCHP addresses multiple dimensions of quality as separate issues in measurement and control.

LEARNING FROM OTHER INDUSTRIES

In mid-1985, when I was asked to take on the job of developing regularized, quantitative, managerially useful systems for measuring and reporting on the quality of care provided by my HMO, I naturally turned first to the health care literature for guidance. Though the literature is deep and often scientifically strong, it is frustrat-ingly devoid of useful tools for managerial action. In my search

207

for help, I turned to additional sources--manufacturers, service industries, high technology firms, and others--and found there is a much richer and deeper discipline for applied quality control. Health care, it seems to me, is several decades behind other industries in its theories and tools for quality measurement and quality improvement; we have much to learn from them.

The technical and scientific foundations for industrial quality control have roots reaching into the early twentieth century, and are grounded largely in applied statistics, operations research, and engineering. With that science has come a set of principles for quality improvement. These principles, first implemented by the Japanese in the mid-twentieth century (though taught to them, ironically, by American thinkers who were being nearly ignored in this country), have offered the Japanese a giant lead on American companies ever since the 1960s.[7]

One such principle is that quality is not introduced by inspection; that no one has ever "inspected" quality into anything. Inspecting final products as a way to assure their quality is the most expensive way to protect the consumer. Imagine a river in which many streams converge, some polluted, some not. Inspection of the final product is, at best, like trying to decrease pollution by treating water at the mouth of the river--expensive, wasteful, and almost certainly incomplete. How much more efficient it might be to move upstream, find feeder streams which contain the pollutants, and intercept the problems before they reach the main river. Modern quality control engineers constantly try to move the quality control process, along with measurement, upstream in the production process.

In fact, for the modern quality control engineer, the ultimate locus upstream is the design of the production process; quality is ultimately a feature of design, not of the product itself. This focus on high-quality design--designs which cannot fail to do what they are intended to do--is one of the most powerful concepts of industrial quality control. Sound designs tend both to reduce costs and to improve quality. The same focus, rare in the health care quality debate, may have much to offer health care. Almost all of today's rhetoric is about inspection of care, and usually at the mouth of the stream. We could benefit enormously--probably both in lower costs and higher quality--by renewing attention to the design of health care systems, which have developed largely by historical accident and not often from contemplation of many alternatives.

An example may help. In a hotel in which I recently stayed, I left a wake-up call at the front desk for 7:00 a.m. Due to a time zone change, however, I awoke at 6:00 a.m., and, unable to fall back to sleep, went out to jog without informing the front desk. I returned at 7:15 a.m. to find a bellhop knocking loudly at my door. I asked him what he was doing. He replied, "You left a wake-up call, and there was no answer when we called. I'm just here to make sure you woke up."

That is what an engineer would call "quality by design." No amount of inspection of performance of the hotel's wake-up call system would ever have been able to improve the quality of performance of that system in the same way that this backup system did. It is a better system--a higher-quality system--because it is designed better, not because it is inspected better.

A second lesson from industry is that quality control must precede cost control. In industry, quality improvement is partially grounded in the notion of the "cost of quality," by which is meant the excess costs in a system of production which result from deficiencies in quality. Such costs include, for example, the costs of inspecting final products to assure their fitness for use, discarding and replacing defective products, revising and controlling production processes, and loss of consumers because of defective goods.

In many industries, these costs of quality can be 50 percent or more of the total cost of goods sold, and efforts to improve quality, especially upstream efforts in design or process control, can yield high multiples of return on the initial investment. One commonly hears from industrial experts stories of a few thousands of dollars invested in a quality control process yielding millions of dollars in production costs downstream, with the simultaneous result of improved products.

No one knows what the costs of quality are in American health care. They may be substantial, but we will not know until we invest in quality improvement as a primary goal. American health care today operates with an extremely high discount rate; it is today's insurance premium level that delivers today's market share. We are consequently underinvesting in the forms of quality improvement that may yield dividends later on in better and more efficient care. If we could learn from industry, we would believe that controlling costs ought to start with improving quality; instead, we insist on the assumption, which has failed many industries, that the problem is to maintain quality while lowering costs. The sequence may be wrong.

A third lesson from industrial quality control is that the worker culture is an absolutely essential ingredient of high quality. One cannot produce high quality with demoralized or fearful workers, at least not in the long run. Quality and fear cannot coexist for long. The search for quality is properly grounded in aspiration, not defense.

That lesson seems lost on many contenders in today's health care debate. From the newspapers, it would appear that the main way to preserve the quality of America's health care system is to find the bad guys and get rid of them. We are on a hunt for bad doctors, bad hospitals, and bad HMOs. That kind of search for deficiency may indeed be needed at some level in an industry which has so long worked in monastic privacy, but in the long run the fear that rhetoric produces will consume more than its share of high quality. In enlightened industries, the search for deficient workers has been replaced by an understanding that good managers appeal to the latent aspirations of the average worker, and that the "customer" and "supplier" must engage in forms of dialogue that recognize their overlapping interests. A vocabulary of trust would help American health care.

If doctors become discouraged about their work, we will pay a dear price in quality. In a service industry--especially in one with a central profession like medicine--the ultimate quality of the work performed inevitably reflects the morale and motivation of the professional. The current rhetoric, fear, surveillance, and shifting of control in health care seem to be leading some physicians to withdraw psychologically from their own work to an extent not common before in health care.[8] The pride of the physician in doctoring is a key element of the quality of our health care system, now and in the future. An atmosphere of fear erodes pride. This threat to quality--the eroding joy of the doctor in the work of doctoring--may be very large indeed.

A fourth lesson from industry is that the goal of quality measurement should be primarily to support continual improvement. When health care producers today talk about such measurement, they tend to focus on ways to demonstrate their current excellence. If we seek to measure only to prove that we are good enough, then we miss a great opportunity. It is better to regard measurement as a tool for improvement, embedded in a complete cycle of improvement.

210

Industrial quality control experts often call that cycle for continuous improvement the "Shewhart cycle," named after one of the founding fathers of quality-control theory, Dr. Walter Shewhart.[9] The cycle for continuous improvement begins with clear definition of the goals, aspirations, or intentions of a person or organization, defines the production process through which those goals are to be sought, and, in that context, creates and uses measurement.

In this context, measurement has two roles. First, designing the measurement is a way to be clear about both goals and process; if one can measure a goal or a process, then (and, in the orthodox view, only then) has one defined it clearly. Second, measurement is used to compare achievements to intentions and to guide the fourth step in the cycle--learning from the measurement and using the knowledge to design improvements. The cycle begins again, with revised goals, processes, and measurements producing new knowledge. The cycle continues without interruption. In this view, quality is not the achievement of a set of criteria. Instead, it is a perpetual process of improvement; "high quality" means "getting better always."

In health care, the notion of "getting better" seems to have taken a back seat to "better not be bad." High quality means, it seems, "good enough to stay out of trouble." That is too low an aspiration to guide an enterprise as important as care of the ill and protection of the well.

The cycle for continuous improvement emphasizes that at least three elements are required to improve quality. First, we must have goals, values, and concepts which guide our intentions. We must be clear about what the purpose of health care (or a health care organization) is. Ideally, that definition is a negotiated one, based on dialogue between those who are purchasing or using care and those who are producing it. Industrial quality control experts sometimes refer to this process as clarifying the "customer-supplier" relationship. The core notion is that in any production process there is always a supplier and one or more customers; quality improvement depends on the supplier's clear understandings about the identity and needs of the customer.

The second essential element is some form of control--the ability to change processes in response to information. Such control can be quite voluntary; the superego of the physician, for example, introduces important controls in health care, controls long valued by the profession. Managed care systems have other types of managerial control as well. They offer the opportunity to redesign care systems in response to new goals or new values.

The third element is information. Clear values and sound control systems can work in concert only when information exists through which to compare intention to performance. Information is a device for improvement.

Health care today increasingly has mechanisms for control, but it is weaker in the other two essentials: values and information. Both need clarification to stand guard effectively over quality.

THE HARVARD COMMUNITY HEALTH PLAN

The goal of quality measurement at HCHP has been to follow industrial models relating measurement with the rest of the system and focusing efforts on improvement, not defense.

The measurement program at HCHP begins with a framework defining both attributes of quality and the target events whose quality is to be measured. Attributes of quality are those characteristics of care that reasonable participants in care (doctors, patients, enrolled populations, managers) value independently. Not all attributes are of equal importance, and not all participants would agree on the importance of any particular attribute relative to the others. Nonetheless, quality, as we conceive it, does have many dimensions, each requiring assessment, control, and continual improvement.

At HCHP, the list of attributes includes two from the classic view of health care quality: health status outcomes and technical processes of care. Outcomes include longevity, reduction of pain, and restoration or preservation of functional status. We can assess, for example, five-year cancer survival rates or functional status in victims of myocardial infarction. By technical process, we mean the ability of the HMO to deliver the processes of care that it intends to deliver. If we decide, based upon the best available evidence, that we intend to measure lipid levels in middle-aged men, one measure of the quality of technical process is the proportion of middle-aged male enrollees who have had such tests performed. Similarly, we specify criteria for and measure the interval between discovery of an abnormal Pap smear and the performance of particular follow-up diagnostic procedures.

In the current uncertainty about efficacy of much of health care, the measurement of technical processes can be vulnerable to criticism. How, for example, do we know that Class III Pap smears *ought* to be followed up within X weeks? The philosophy of measurement of technical process is only partially based on assumed connections to health status outcomes. What we really mean to measure in this domain is the ability of the health care system to deliver what it intends to deliver, no matter how those intentions were formed. It is, of course, important that intentions be formed conscientiously and intelligently, but that is a separate issue.

Other attributes of quality are less commonly stressed in research. They include access (the ability of patients to reach care when they feel the need), interpersonal behavior, and the characteristics of our physical plant. These dimensions of quality are often mentioned in the health services research literature as "extra" characteristics, or epiphenomena, of care--of interest to the assessor of quality only to the extent that they are known to be connected to health status outcomes. At HCHP, we include these performance domains in the definition of quality. The patients' sense of being cared *about,* for example, is valued not because of its connection to health status, but because given our organization's values, it ought to be an attribute of the care we give. It stands on its own as a dimension of quality.

One other dimension of particular importance in the HMO is the integration of care, which means mainly the capacity to move information around in service of the patient. An HMO is a complex organism which creates its own hazards. Keeping care for the individual patient organized, smoothly flowing, and coordinated is a challenge in quality control; measuring such integration is an essential part of meeting that challenge. Here we measure, for example, the instances in which primary care physicians are notified in advance of elective surgery to be performed on one of their patients.

The targets of measurement are usually encounters in our HMO. The encounter is an accessible event and a sensible unit to be assessed. In the long run, however, it would be better for an HMO to use some population-based target, such as studying care of enrollees rather than care during visits. The theoretically correct question for an HMO to ask about its own quality is not so much "How did we do in this visit?" but rather "How well are we doing for this group of enrollees?"

Measurement occurs at the intersection of targets and attributes of quality, and each intersection may require its own mode of measurement. Quality measurement at HCHP is an eclectic enterprise, using many different tools, some borrowed directly from other industries. Record review is a mainstay, of course, as in any health care quality assurance effort. But, we also make use of prospective data bases, simulations, probes, patient surveys, testing situations, and direct observation of care. Of these, the most difficult, but in the long run the most promising, are simulations. If one wishes to know how a process is performing, there is no more direct route to measurement than using the process in action. Common use of simulations in health care will require more trust than we have at present, and better techniques for believable simulations, modeled, for example, on the imaginative technologies now used to assess the skills of airline pilots.

Measurement reports emerge steadily from the Department of Quality-of-Care Measurement at HCHP to help devise more efficient methods of display so that managers and clinicians easily can consume technically complex results. Reports are assembled annually into a "State of the Plan" report on quality to the Board of Directors, highlighting areas of strong and weak performance and helping set priorities for managerial action and the redesign of systems. The 1987 report filled two volumes and totalled nearly 150 pages, posing formidable challenges for efficient and easily accessible display of findings.

One key step in the process of continual improvement at HCHP has been to identify areas of special hazard. Where will our performance most likely fail to match our intentions? It is efficient, once these hazard areas have been identified, to focus both measurement and repair on them, moving as far upstream as possible in the production process.

Four hazard areas have emerged: access, communication, responsibility, and skills of nonclinician staff. In an HMO, access can be withheld inadvertently through faulty design of scheduling and telephone systems. Communication among physicians, different clinic sites, and staff specialists is a key component of high quality in a large organization and can be placed at risk as the complexity of the HMO grows with its size. Responsibility for the patient can also become blurred in a large system without fee-for-service incentives; and a safe HMO will take special pains to assure that responsibility in patient management is clearly placed at all times. Finally, the support staff in a complex organization play a key role in assuring the quality of care. Support staff members must be offered the training and ongoing supervision they require, or quality in several of its dimensions will suffer.

An example from one hazard area (access) may help illustrate the complete cycle of improvement. Investigation of a serious complaint from an HMO member suggested that delays between the detection of a suspicious breast lump and a definitive biopsy could be unacceptably long. Discussions between medical managers and surgical staff established more detailed specifications for scheduling biopsies. The Department of Quality-of-Care Measurement was asked to monitor the actual waiting times. The measurements documented excessive variability in referral intervals, which led the managers involved to redesign the referral procedures and to develop and publish an algorithm to guide primary care physicians in the correct sequence of investigations. The improvement process will not end there, however; repeated monitoring will lead to further redesign if needed, and the measurement will also include careful patient surveys to determine if technical specifications meet the needs of the patients.

What may distinguish the measurement processes in this vignette from the more common form of quality assurance in health care is this: the clients for whom the measurements were conducted were the medical managers in HCHP, and the measurements were intended to help the system improve, not to defend the system from external accusations. The first question asked of any quality measurement process in HCHP is, "Who is the client?" The answer to this question determines the data to be included in the report and made in its presentation.

In health care, we are just beginning to devise useful responses to the demand for information on quality within and outside organizations. It may be too soon for purchasers and users of care to expect that the results of these nascent measurements will be useful and comparable among organizations. A better question may be this: How can one tell whether a health care organization is really serious about improving, instead of simply engaging in defensive measurement to protect itself against the demands for information from outsiders? The following may be useful as predicates of effective quality control and, therefore, as signals of serious intent in a health care producer to gain control of quality.

Quality control must be grounded in values; it must be based on aspiration. Organizations that wish to improve their quality must know what they value and share a sense of common purpose throughout their ranks. Quality improvement cannot be based upon defense. In the current health care marketplace, the values espoused by an organization increasingly are the products of negotiation with consumers. High-quality health care organizations, therefore, must have systems in place which permit them to listen to and engage in dialogue with their consumers.

Quality improvement must begin with commitment at the very top of the organization. To know how effective an organization is likely to be in improving quality, find out where quality measurement and quality assurance report in the organization. If the quality assurance office is down the street in rented space and headed by a lower level manager, it is unlikely that the organization is truly committed to quality improvement. It is probably more interested in proving than in improving its quality.

Quality improvement takes money. Examine the budget of the quality measurement function in a health care organization. Asked for that information, many organizations will tell how much they spend on utilization review, and call it quality measurement. Utilization review is not quality measurement, and it is not quality control. At present, it may be reasonable for HMO plan purchasers to begin to expect that as much as one-half of 1 percent of their health care premium dollar should be spent on measuring quality. To repeat, this figure is not to include utilization review costs.

Organizations committed to quality improvement will have mechanisms for horizontal integration of quality measurement and control up and down the line of management. At any level, down to the front line, staff should regard the quality measurement function as relevant to them and useful in their work. Measuring for improvement is a theme in high-quality work cultures. In health care, measurement must include the participation of quality measurement professionals at organization-wide meetings. In its analysis of the space shuttle Challenger accident, the Presidential commission investigating the causes concluded, in part, that failure "to get critical information to the proper levels of management" was a key factor.[10] Unless quality measurement staff regularly are present in managerial meetings, such failures are virtually inevitable, and measurement is likely to become irrelevant to internal decisions.

Organizing to improve quality requires statistical sophistication. Quality measurement is a science which must be taught and learned. In organizations committed to improvement, one finds a statistically skilled individual at a high level supervising the dissemination of skills and measurement techniques throughout the organization.

To achieve continual improvement, managers must constantly refocus attention on design, not simply on performance. In health care, as in other industries, the highest quality will be achieved by those organizations that invest in continual analysis and experimentation in the design of care systems and processes. In effect, the old saying "If it ain't broke, don't fix it" is a poor guide to quality improvement. The guiding idea is "There must be a way to make it better."

In improving quality, there is no substitute for responsive management. Without managers who remove obstacles to improvement, quality will decay. To find high quality in an HMO, look for managers who can listen and fix something. An internal emphasis on grades, performance reviews, and employee discipline is far less indicative of high quality than are managers known by their employees to be ready to help them get their jobs done.

Finally, to find quality, look for an organization with a corporate strategy to drive out fear. Reactive postures, a focus on discipline, an environment of surveillance--these are not elements of real quality improvement. Indeed, if the health-care industry as a whole regards quality measurement mainly as a burden laid upon it by an unwise or insatiable outside force, quality will not improve. If the purchasers of health care services regard quality measurement as a search for a deficient few, quality will not improve. If instead both purchasers and producers of health care can understand quality measurement as a necessary tool for improving our capacity to do what health care exists to do--to help people in pain, calm those in fear, and save those in peril--if we look at quality measurement as a step on the route to improvement, then quality can improve.

NOTES

1. K. McPherson, J.E. Wennberg, O.B. Hovind, and P. Clifford, "Small-Area Variations in the Use of Common Surgical Procedures: An International Comparison of New England, England, and Norway," *New England Journal of Medicine,* 307 (1982): 1310-1314.

2. J.E. Wennberg and A. Gittelsohn, "Variations in Medical Care Among Small Areas," *Scientific American,* 246 (1982): 120-133.

3. D.M. Berwick and K.C. Coltin, "Feedback Reduces Test Use in a Health Maintenance Organization," *Journal of the American Medical Association,* 255 (1986): 1450-1454.

4. B. Payne, T. Lyons, L. Dwarshius, M. Kolton, and W. Morris, *The Quality of Medical Care: Evaluation and Improvement* (Chicago: Hospital Research and Educational Trust, 1976).

5. R.H. Brook, K.N. Williams, and A.D. Avery. "Quality Assurance Today and Tomorrow: Forecast for the Future," *Annals of Internal Medicine,* 85 (1976): 809-817.

6. J.W. Williamson, *Assessing and Improving Health Care Outcomes: The Health Accounting Approach to Quality Assurance* (Cambridge, MA: Ballinger, 1978).

7. H.M. Wadsworth, K.S. Stephens, and A.B. Godfrey, *Modern Methods for Quality Control and Improvement* (New York: John Wiley & Sons, 1986).

8. R. Berrien, "What Future for Primary Care Private Practice?" *New England Journal of Medicine,* 316 (1987): 334-337.

9. W.E. Deming, *Out of the Crisis* (Cambridge, MA: MIT Press, 1986).

10. *Report by the Presidential Commission on the Space Shuttle Challenger Accident* (Washington, DC: U.S. Government Printing Office, 1986).

Chapter 11

The Quality of Nursing Home Care: The Institute of Medicine's Blueprint for its Improvement

Karl D. Yordy

The quality of care in nursing homes has been the focus of increasing attention from policymakers and the public. This attention derives from the rapid growth in the elderly population (from whom come the bulk of nursing home residents), repeated findings of inadequate care in many nursing homes despite regulatory efforts to eliminate such care, and the inherent difficulties in defining and assuring the quality of care for these frail and vulnerable individuals.

The Institute of Medicine (IOM) of the National Academy of Sciences recently completed a far-reaching study of nursing home quality that produced a comprehensive blueprint for reform of the regulation of quality in nursing home care.[1] The study was carried out by a distinguished committee appointed by the IOM and representing many different perspectives on nursing home care, including persons with research expertise related to nursing home care, operators of nursing homes in both the for-profit and not-for-profit sectors, consumer advocates, persons experienced in administration of federal and state regulatory programs, and health professionals and health services researchers addressing the problems of an aging society. The study was supported by the federal government to help resolve continuing disagreement among federal policymakers concerning directions for the improvement of regulation of nursing homes.

Before summarizing the committee's plan for improving quality, a few observations about the nature of the nursing home enterprise will make clear the challenges inherent in assuring quality in this important health care setting:

1). Nursing homes are big business in the U.S. In 1985, there were 15,000 nursing homes with 1.5 million beds certified for the care of Medicaid and Medicare patients.

2). Seventy percent of nursing homes with 80 percent of the beds are owned by for-profit organizations.

3). Occupancy rates are high--well over 90 percent in most states.

4). Profound demographic changes are fueling the demand for nursing home care. In 1985, there were 2.85 million Americans over 85. By the year 2000 that number will increase to 5.1 million--an 80 percent increase in 15 years. If current patterns are followed, one out of five persons over 85 will be in a nursing home. The demand may increase further because pressures to reduce hospitalization will result in additional patients being referred for nursing home care. These patients tend to be sicker patients, requiring more nursing home services.

5). Almost 50 percent of expenditures for nursing home care come from the Medicaid program. Medicare is a very small factor, with about 2 percent of the expenditures. Seventy percent of patients within a given year have some or all of their care paid for by Medicaid.

6). Whereas quality of care in hospitals is generally perceived to be good, quality of care in many nursing homes has been found deficient in study after study over the past 15 years.

7). Most nursing home occupants are residents as well as patients; that is, the nursing home is their place of residence, not just a place where they receive care. Therefore, quality of life is an important aspect of the overall quality of care in nursing homes.

8). Nursing home care is regulated directly by state agencies under federal standards and guidelines. There is no delegation of regulatory review to private organizations, such as deemed status for review of hospital care under the Medicare program by the Joint Commission on Accreditation of Healthcare Organizations.

Turning now to the IOM study, the central findings were that: 1) despite substantial improvements in the quality of care rendered by nursing homes in the United States over the last decade or so, there continues to be far too many instances of grossly inadequate care; and 2) that the general level of quality in nursing homes is not as high as it could and should be.[2] Further, it was the clear and explicit conclusion of the committee that, given the history of the nursing home industry and of the regulation of nursing homes, and given the characteristics of the nursing home market, it is imperative that regulatory activities be strengthened and improved, especially at the federal level. While "deregulation" may be the trend in transportation or communications, it is clearly inappropriate for nursing homes given past experience, current market character-istics, and the extent of government involvement in, and obligation to, nursing home residents.[3]

Since 1974, a regulatory process for nursing homes has been in place. It was established by federal standards and requirements but is administered by the states. This regulatory process focuses on the *capacity* of nursing homes to provide quality care, not on the care given or the outcomes of that care. Thus, it has largely been aimed at the structure of care, rather than its processes or outcomes. For example, it has been possible to certify an institution for participation in Medicare and Medicaid without seeing a patient. The IOM committee recommended a complete reorientation of this regulatory approach to make it patient-centered and outcome-oriented.

At the heart of this new approach would be a standardized resident assessment system. The committee recommended that all nursing homes be required to make standard assessments of all residents on admission, and periodically thereafter, and to record the data in a standard way in the official medical record.[4] Standard resident assessment data across facilities would establish norms that currently are not available. The data would include descriptions of services and the degree of well-being for residents who have similar characteristics. This resident assessment data would give inspectors an objective basis for comparing quality of care and the functional aspects of quality of life. More effective and valid regulation would be facilitated, and a powerful means for identifying deficient nursing homes would be provided.

Such assessment also would give nursing home managers a useful tool that most do not now have. Competent assessment of each resident's functional, medical, mental, and social status is essential to plan a care program which is individually tailored to the resident's needs. Moreover, the introduction of this system is likely to have a positive effect on the attitudes and behavior of nursing home staff at all levels. Resident assessment data would also provide a basis for an objective analysis of the effects of different patterns of care or different resource uses. Therefore, it should contribute to the efficiency of nursing home care.

The committee recommended abolishing the current distinctions between skilled nursing facilities (SNFs) and intermediate care facilities (ICFs) on the grounds that, in practical application, these distinctions have little meaning. The range of differences among the states in the proportions of care provided in SNFs or ICFs is very wide. For example, in Arizona, all nursing homes are SNFs; in Oklahoma 98 percent are ICFs.[5] A single standard of care should apply. This single classification would have the practical effect of raising care standards for many ICFs, such as requiring supervision of nursing aides by skilled registered nurses. These changes could have the effect of raising costs in some locations, but the committee felt those costs would be justified by the higher standards.

Because nursing home residents often live in nursing homes for extended periods of time, and because they are often frail or confused, the committee emphasized the need to include quality-of-life standards among the nursing home performance criteria and to give additional emphasis to residents' rights. The committee also recommended prohibiting discrimination against residents supported by Medicaid, increasing social service staffing, and training nurse's aides who provide most of the care.

The committee recommended a number of changes in the processes used to monitor care. These include:

1). Flexible timing of surveys to make them less predictable; and

2). A two-stage survey process to focus attention where it is needed most, with a first survey as a screen for deficiencies, followed by a more intensive second survey when needed.

In addition to better performance criteria, a new source of data, and improvements in the survey process, the committee made a number of recommendations to improve the enforcement of regulatory standards. The committee based these recommendations on the ample evidence that enforcement is needed to assure quality of care. Under the current approach, the primary enforcement tool is decertification. Decertification is an "atom bomb" approach to sanctions, with the effects falling on innocent nursing home residents as much as, or more than, on the nursing home owner. The committee recommended that the Medicaid statute be amended to authorize a standard set of intermediate sanctions that could be used by both state and federal governments. These intermediate sanctions would include a ban on admissions, civil fines, receiverships, and emergency authority to close facilities and transfer residents. Authority to impose severe sanctions on chronic violators also would be provided. The committee estimated that perhaps 10 to 15 percent of facilities fall into the category of repeat violators. Present statutory authority is not adequate to deal with these facilities. Moreover, for the really bad facilities, the law should be amended to make the appeals process on sanctions less attractive.

While effective regulation is essential, it is not sufficient to insure adequate quality of care and quality of life in nursing homes. Other important factors are: 1) consumer involvement; 2) community involvement within nursing homes; 3) positive motivation and technical competence of ownership, management, and staff; and 4) a professional climate that will attract highly motivated, ethical, and well-qualified staff.

The committee recommended that the Ombudsman Program, which is authorized by the Older Americans Act of 1978, be strengthened both by amending the legislation and by recommending that the Administration on Aging, Department of Health and Human Services, give it much stronger and more effective leadership.[6] The Ombudsman Program provides a statutory basis for the role of consumer advocacy. Consumer advocacy plays an important role in quality assurance in nursing homes because residents are a particularly vulnerable group, and nursing home regulators are only occasional visitors to nursing homes. Ombudsmen investigate and resolve complaints, provide information to public agencies about problems that nursing home residents have experienced, and provide training for staff and volunteers. The statue is broad, local programs vary widely, and funding is inadequate. The committee's recommendations were aimed at providing a more substantial foundation for these important functions. The committee also offered suggestions in other areas, including introduction of incentives for rewarding consistently high quality care, for example, preference to institutions with good records when awarding certificates-of-need for constructing new facilities or expanding existing ones.

Finally, the committee identified issues that need further study. These included the following: 1) the scope and design of information systems needed to regulate nursing homes effectively and facilitate development of sound policies for long-term care; 2) policies governing the method and amount of payment to nursing homes for care of residents eligible for support under the Medicaid program; 3) policies affecting the supply of nursing home beds in the context of the growing demand for all types of long-term care services; 4) regulatory policies concerning the training and qualifications of all staff in nursing homes; 5) minimum staffing patterns needed to provide adequate care; and 6) policies governing construction for new nursing homes, specifically the proportion of single rooms that should be required.

The committee believed very strongly that an improved regulatory process, as detailed in its report, is absolutely necessary to maintain and improve the quality of care and the quality of life for nursing home residents. Such regulation will make a difference in the quality of nursing home care. This position was the unanimous view of a diverse committee and was agreed to despite the current trend in public policy toward deregulation and greater dependence on market forces.

The model of quality assurance that would be in place if all of these recommendations were adopted would have the following characteristics--many of which may be instructive for quality assurance in other aspects of health care:

1). A broad definition of quality, leading to criteria that include those characteristics of care seen as important by the patient, as well as characteristics deemed important from the provider's perspective.

2). An outcome-orientation that focuses on the results of care, rather than what goes into that care.

3). A method for generating objective data about outcomes that can be used to monitor care, to improve internal operating efficiencies, and to improve our knowledge about performance criteria.

4). Mechanisms for public oversight consistent with the long tradition of a public responsibility for assuring those aspects of quality that cannot be easily monitored by individuals themselves, and consistent with the need to assure the appropriate use of the substantial public funds being provided for this care.

5). Sanctions for poor performance that are appropriate for the specific problem.

The committee's scope did not include the relationship between methods of payment, cost containment, and the quality of care. These issues loom large for nursing homes just as they do for hospital care. Under the Medicaid program, payment amounts and mechanisms for payment for nursing home care vary widely from state to state, and Medicaid, as stated above, is the dominant payment source in most states. The committee observed, however, that while the relationship of payment to quality deserves further study, there are good and bad nursing homes in low-payment states and good and bad nursing homes in high-payment states. It was thus apparent to the committee that an objective means to monitor care and appropriate sanctions for poor performance were necessary regardless of the methods and amounts of payment.

CONCLUSION

This paper summarizes the essence of the committee's conclusions and detailed recommendations (forty-five in number). An unusual degree of agreement has been reached between consumer advocates, the nursing home industry, and state officials concerning the desired implementation of these recommendations.[7] As a result, the report has received substantial attention from policymakers in both the legislative and executive branches. Many of these recommendations were enacted into law in late 1987.[8] In January 1988, the Health Care Financing Administration (HCFA) published regulatory changes that implement many of the remaining recommendations that could be carried out through administrative action.[9] HCFA had previously noted that some of the committee's recommendations continued to rely on structure and process measures, rather than outcome measures.[10] In the committee's view, however, these structural standards of care are a necessary transition phase between the current regulatory system and a future system based on the availability and use of objective resident assessment data. These data can, in turn, provide objective criteria against which one can measure the influence of the structure and the process of care on its outcomes.

The directions set by the committee are clear, and a firm agenda for action has been provided. The above regulatory changes and the legislative changes proposed by Congress will be major steps in implementing the agenda. The result will be a more objective, patient-centered, and enforceable system of regulation that will improve and maintain the quality of care in nursing homes.

NOTES

1. Institute of Medicine, *Improving the Quality of Care in Nursing Homes* (Washington, DC: National Academy Press, March 1986).

2. Ibid., p. 3.

3. Ibid., pp. 4-5.

4. Ibid., pp. 74-77.

5. Ibid., p. 72.

6. U.S. Congress, Older Americans Act of 1965 as amended in 1984 (Washington, DC: U.S. Government Printing Office, 1985).

7. U.S. Senate, Subcommittee on Health of the Committee on Finance, April 28, 1987.

8. Public Law 100-203, Section 4201-4218.

9. Final regulations published in the *Federal Register*, January 14, 1988.

10. U.S., Senate, Subcommittee on Health of the Committee on Finance, April 28, 1987, statement by William Roper, M.D., Administrator, Health Care Financing Administration.

Chapter 12

Quality Assurance and Medical Education

Ruth M. Covell, M.D.

A commonly voiced problem in hospital corridors and Peer Review Organizations (PROs) is how to get even a bare-bones cadre of physicians to participate in quality assurance (QA) activities. In the fifteen years since the inception of the federally sponsored patient care review programs (first Professional Standards Review Organizations and now PROs), there has been no substantial improvement in this situation. Nonetheless, an increased willingness by physicians to participate in QA activities in the future can be anticipated as a result of three converging forces:

1). An improvement in the perception of the relevance of the review process to the everyday practice of physicians;

2). The increasing credibility of the review process gained by improvements in review methodology and the use of standards based on both sound research and "consensus conferences"; and

3). Developments in medical education and the organization of health care which are contributing to a physician readiness to accept and participate in review activities.

This chapter will focus on the third area mentioned--the medical education community, which can increase its contribution to the quality assurance effort in three ways:

1). By developing programs, activities, and an environment which favorably shape the attitudes of physicians and other health care professionals towards the need for quality assurance programs and which motivate them to participate in such programs;

229

2). By providing physicians-in-training with the technical skills necessary to participate comfortably and effectively in review activities; and

3). By stimulating, in a subset of trainees, an interest in research issues germane to the improvement of quality assurance programs.

ATTITUDE ADJUSTMENT

Data suggest that some progress is being made regarding attitudes towards peer review, but a lot still remains to be accomplished. A recent survey of more than 600 randomly selected California physicians, conducted by the Bureau of Research and Planning of the California Medical Association, solicited opinions on a variety of current medical socioeconomic issues.[1] Included were several questions related to quality assurance. As Table 1 clearly indicates, there are significant differences of opinion among the physician respondents based on both age and sex.

Of particular interest is the response to the statement: "Quality of care is a professional responsibility; government has no role in establishing standards or criteria to assess the quality of care provided to patients by physicians." Overall, almost 60 percent of the responding physicians agreed that the government should not have a role in establishing standards for quality of care. Concurrence fell to 51 percent, however, among physicians under the age of 50, and only 31 percent of women physicians agreed with the statement. A difference by specialty was also apparent. Almost 68 percent of surgical specialists agreed with the statement, compared to 52 percent of medical specialists.

Reaction to the second quality-related statement, "Outside peer review organizatons are an unnecessary imposition on my professional judgment and autonomy," was even more striking. Only 37.6 percent of physicians under age 40 agreed with this statement, while 57.6 percent of physicians in the 50- to 59-year-old age category agreed. Again, women stood out. Only 27 percent agreed with the statement, compared to over 53 percent of the men. There was no significant difference in response by specialty area.

There are several possible explanations for the variation observed by age category. One is that the variation is a function of more experience changing one's view regarding peer review organizations. However, the findings suggest a different scenario. Younger physicians are being trained and are coming into practice in a health care world markedly different from that of less than a generation ago. The majority of young physicians are electing to practice in group or institutional settings in which the observance of organizational rules, regulations, and standards is commonplace, and individual autonomy is somewhat sacrificed. When the survey results were analyzed by practice arrangement, fee-for-service physicians were most likely to agree with the statements. In other words, they view peer organizations more negatively. These factors probably account for the significant differences in the response by female physicians, because they are generally younger and, in even greater numbers than men, elect salaried practice settings. As the proportion of women physicians, as well as the proportion of physicians in managed practice settings, increases, physician resistance to external peer review and to the consensual building of standards of care will most likely continue to erode.

The responses to two additional questions on the survey are noteworthy. Men and women generally responded similarly to the statement: "To assure continuing competence, physicians should be periodically examined and relicensed." Slightly over half concur with the statement, but with startling differences by age. Over 69 percent of those under 40 agreed with the statement, compared to 43 percent of those in the 50- to 59-year-old category. This finding again may be a reflection of the fact that younger physicians are establishing their practices at a time when they expect to be subjected to more external controls and ongoing evaluation of their professional competency.

The final statement of interest is: "Since it is obviously impossible for any one person to know all about medicine today, specialty licensure would be good idea." About 20 percent of the physicians expressed no opinion on the statement. Of those with an opinion, half agreed. Not surprisingly, general and family practitioners were much less favorably disposed to this approach to quality control, presumably because of perceived restrictions on the scope of their practices.

The responses cited above demonstrate that the changing milieu of clinical practice and the expectations of young physicians will have a strong influence on physician acceptance of quality assurance programs in the future. The positive attitudes of the younger physicians illustrated could also be a function of recent changes in medical education. We will discuss these new educational initiatives below. As the young cohort of physicians matures, it will ultimately comprise the majority of the practitioners. It will be important to monitor over time the attitudes of these physicians, as well as those of even newer physicians, to estimate the impact on them of experience and the changes in medical education.

MEDICAL EDUCATION AND QUALITY ASSURANCE ATTITUDES AND SKILLS

Medical schools and other health professional schools can play an important role in speeding up the evolution in physician attitudes towards, and involvement in, quality assurance by teaching the skills which underlie the quality assurance review process. Anecdotal information indicates that quality assurance presently is not dealt with in more than a passing way in other than a few medical schools. Despite the enthusiasm of a small cadre of faculty members, this deficiency may not improve substantially in the near future, owing to the pressures of an already crowded curriculum and the status of quality assurance activities among medical school decision makers. There are, however, several developments in undergraduate medical education that would appear to be important in better preparing physicians for the analytical rigors of good QA efforts and for self-evaluation of their own practice.

First, virtually all schools now cover what could be considered the basic sciences of quality assurance: statistics, epidemiology, ethics, and, to a lesser extent, other social and behavioral sciences. A recent addition to this list of covered topics is the application of the principles of decision analysis to patient care. While this application is still in the embryonic stages of development, it is beginning to take hold in a number of medical schools as faculty members develop specific expertise in the field, and students increasingly are introduced to elective and sometimes required courses in the field.

In a nutshell, medical decision analysis attempts to provide a logical approach to common clinical problems when the results of decisions cannot be foretold with a high degree of certainty.[2] In decision analysis, the medical process is represented by a decision tree. Probabilities of certain actions are introduced, and the outcomes of each action must be specified. The patient can be brought into the process by expressing preferences for various outcomes. Although there is debate about whether individual physicians should become adept at decision analysis or whether they should simply be able to intelligently interpret analysis performed by experts, its use will focus attention on decision making in clincial practice and thus enhance quality assurance review and interest.

A second important development that should lead to improved interests and skill in patient care assessment is the explicit attention now being devoted in medical education to the development, management, and use of self-generated clinical data bases and to the identificiation, access, and use of clinical data bases that are in the public domain. These educational advances should have a profound impact on the involvement of physicians in quality assurance activities ten to twenty years hence, as physicians acquire the skills to take advantage of technological advances in evaluating not only the current progress and short-range outcomes of patient care, but also the expected longer range health status and needs of their patients.

Despite these advances, there is no consensus as to what would be ideal in terms of content and sequencing of quality assurance efforts in medical education. During the first two years, many schools provide courses, or devote portions thereof, to medical ethics, human values, and health care delivery issues. In these courses, students are introduced to the historical basis of medical practice and the rapid changes now taking place in the financing and organization of health care. In a required course that I teach in the second year at the University of California, San Diego, quality assurance is introduced both as an individual physician's responsibility and as the profession's responsibility to the public at large. An introduction to organized quality assurance programs is also included.

This type of course, as well as courses on ethics and values which emphasize small group discussions and student presentations, in addition to lectures, generates lively debates on the cost of medical care, the marginal effectiveness of interventions, and quality tradeoffs. Students come to understand the need for vigilance over the quality of care in the face of the increasing financial and organization incentives on all fronts to reduce services. The positive and negative impacts on quality of care of surpluses and shortages of health care practitioners, in both geographic and speciality areas, is also debated.

When this course was first offered, students began to actually challenge the faculty about its curriculum content and introduce their own topics and approaches as they progressed through their third and fourth year clerkships. In the last few years, however, due mainly to the new-found prominence of these issues within the professional societies, the faculty is catching up with the students. Unfortunately, at other schools many such courses are elective or, worse still, quality assurance content is missing altogether.

In clerkship training, goals are increasingly being set by the faculty to address: 1) the need for an appreciation of the importance of research on, and the evaluation of, medical practices; 2) the need for physicians to evaluate their own practice style; and 3) the need to revise concepts, knowledge, and skills as necessary. A few newer and more clinically oriented schools include, among other techniques, explicit QA instruction by means of mock QA committees, QA material in case conferences, and exposure to physicians involved in QA programs.[3] Several institutions have been successful in introducing electives in the fourth year which return, with more of a clinical focus, to the concepts of quality assurance and ethics that were touched on during the first two years. In most schools, however, cost consciousness, to the extent it is being taught at all, is still being addressed more than concern for quality of care.

At the house staff level, residents are now being trained in an environment in which quality assurance activities are a way of life. The particular institution's commitment to quality assurance and the attitudes of the physician faculty involved will influence an individual resident's attitudes; this attitude will carry over into early years of practice. If these attitudes are not positive, compliance with the "mechanics" of the review activities may be seen as an intrusion on the resident's time devoted to direct patient care, rather than a process which enhances care if handled thoughtfully.

Some programs, such as the internal medicine program at the University of Vermont, build quality control activities into the day-to-day experience of the residents.[4] The knowledge of patient care outcomes and other information generated through these quality assurance activities are used as an aid in identifying the individual training needs of each resident. The cost of tests and procedures ordered by the residents in this program places them at the 20 percentile level for all trainees. The residents' performance on specialty boards, however, is consistently above the 90th percentile level (which, one would hope, correlates somewhat with better patient care!). This experience suggests an ideal marriage of quality assurance, cost containment activities, and educational objectives--and the direction QA activities involving practicing physicians should take. Unfortunately, most educational initiatives at the undergraduate and graduate medical levels that involve "hands on" clinical work do not, to date, include exposure to the use of aggregate data in analyzing practice profiles, setting objectives for groups of patients, or analyzing outcomes.

A discussion of quality assurance in medical education would not be complete without mentioning continuing education. Incorporation of quality assurance into broadly based, discipline-oriented continuing education has the potential of reaching a very broad audience. Unfortunately, most continuing education programs on quality assurance entail the converted lecturing to the equally knowledgeable. Much can be gained by encouraging physicians new to the QA effort to simply "dig in and get dirty." In this area, there is still a role for the "see one, do one, teach one" principle of medical education.

QUALITY ASSURANCE RESEARCH

The third challenge to medical schools is to excite students to the many opportunities for research relating to quality assurance. This challenge is met in some institutions by offering to medical students independent study opportunities and to residents the opportunity for clinical research projects. The latter opportunity occurs particularly in the primary care specialties.

Incorporating the opportunity into advanced residency and fellowship training in such fields as internal medicine and geriatrics, as well as family medicine, would appear critical to the development of future faculty members with an interest in quality assurance. The Robert Wood Johnson Clinical Scholars Program has begun to address this need. A substantive introduction to research related to quality assurance at an earlier level of training is necessary, however, if a significant number of future investigators is to emerge. A positive future scenario for enhanced physician involvement in quality assurance research is also dependent on enhanced federal support for both health services research, the academic field underlying quality assurance, and clinical research.

More direct involvement of medical schools in quality assurance research using the expertise and data developed by review programs would be beneficial to the schools' education and research missions and to the "practicing" quality assurance community. For the most part, medical school faculty have not played leadership roles in PROs, and many practicing physicians would probably like to keep it that way. Nonetheless, the level of sophisticiation now achieved, and the substantial data now being generated, in the QA field all but demand linkages between PROs and medical schools in order to reap the maximum analytical benefit from the data collected.

The social loss of not taking advantage of the data in hand could be great. Current budgets of the review organizations simply do not allow the type of data base exploration that may be possible in a research environment. Another spinoff of such relationships would be the involvement of students and the promotion of the next generation of quality assurance investigators. Barriers between the two types of organizations need to be broken down. Medical school investigators need to stop looking at the review data as being too dirty to touch, and the review organizations need to recognize that the hassels of becoming involved with educational institutions have long-term payoffs in meeting their own objectives, as well as those of the larger quality assurance effort.

CONCLUSION

Developments in the physician practice environment suggest a more favorable attitude toward quality assurance by practicing physicians in the future. Medical education holds the promise of both furthering this attitude of change and of providing future physicians with the conceptual base and technical skills necessary for successful quality assurance programs. Medical education also has the opportunity to prepare future investigators for research in quality assurance. Substantive progress in attaining these goals has important implications both for the quality of patient care during the many years in which physicians are in training, as well as during their subsequent practices, and for enhancing the quality assurance research agenda.

Table 1

Level of Agreement of Practicing Physicians With Statements About Medical Quality Assurance, by Specialty, Sex and Age*

Statement	Percent in Agreement	GP/FP	Medical	Surgical	Other	Male	Female	Less than 40	40-49	50-59	60 & Over
"Quality of care is a professional responsibility; government has no role in establishing standards or criteria to assess the quality of care provided to patients by physicians."	59.9%	65.2%	52.4%	67.7%	54.4%	61.8%	30.8%	51.1%	64.5%	60.8%	58.6%
"Outside peer review organizations are an unnecessary imposition on my professional judgment and autonomy." 53.4%	50.1%	53.9%	50.0%	54.3%		44.4%	53.4%	26.9%	37.6%	50.7%	56.6%
"To assure continuing competence, physicians should be periodically re-examined and relicensed."	51.7%	58.4%	54.1%	49.4%	48.3%	50.9%	53.8%	69.2%	47.4%	43.4%	49.4%
"Since it is obviously impossible for any one person to learn everything about medicine today, specialty licensure would be a good idea."	47.8%	38.2%	51.8%	47.0%	49.4%	47.2%	46.2%	50.4%	46.7%	49.7%	45.4%

*Adapted from California Medical Association, Bureau of Research and Planning, "Socioeconomic Report," 26(Oct./Nov. 1986).

NOTES

1. Bureau of Research and Planning, California Medical Association, "Socioeconomic Report," vol. XXVI, no.7 (October/November 1986).

2. S.G. Parker and J.P. Kassiner, "Decision Analysis," *New England Journal of Medicine,* 316(1987): 250-258.

3. J.W. Williamson, *Teaching Quality Assurance and Cost Containment in Health Care* (San Francisco, CA: Jossey-Bass Publishers, 1982).

4. R.E. Bouchard, H.M. Tufo, and H.N. Beaty, "The Impact of a Quality Assurance Program on Postgraduate Training in Internal Medicine," *Journal of the American Medical Association,* 253(1985): 1146-1150.

Chapter 13

Quality Health Care in a Cost-Conscious Environment: The Intervention of Third-Party Payers in Determining Medical Necessity and the Changing Rights and Liabilities of Health Care Practitioners*

Barry J. London, J.D., and Leslie B. Harris, J.D.

In many people's eyes, cost containment or utilization review is the bad brother of quality assurance in health care. That view is based on the belief that any restriction on expenditures results in compromised health care to the detriment of the patient. However, cost containment, which is achieved by limiting the utilization of medical resources, need not be viewed as an impediment to quality health care.

First, cost containment programs are aimed only at avoiding excessive expenditures. Second, by avoiding waste and reducing expenses, third-party payers are more likely to have funds available to provide services when they are needed. In short, since insurers' resources are finite, cost containment is a prerequisite to the survival of medical insurance programs and the delivery of insured health care.

As a result of the introduction of cost-containment programs, third-party payers have entered into the medical decision-making arena. Once heralded as a sacred place for the treating physician, courts have held that government, private medical insurers, and peer review organizations are at liberty to determine whether or not the treatment rendered to an individual was "medically necessary" and therefore within the scope of coverage. The intervention of third-party payers in the decision-making process introduces new actors into the field of liability. As the following cases demonstrate, however, courts have refused to shift the ultimate responsibility for negligent decisions from the patient's physician to the payer.

---

*Copyright held by the authors.

239

RETROSPECTIVE REVIEW

One method used by third-party reviewers to determine whether the care rendered by a physician or hospital was "medically necessary" is retrospective review. In retrospective review, the third party's determination is made after the care is rendered and thus has no bearing on the care that is actually rendered. Disagreement with the physician or hospital merely triggers a fight over money.[1]

The retrospective method of review was recently challenged by a beneficiary in *Sarchett v. Blue Shield of California*.[2] The beneficiary claimed that Blue Shield's practice of retrospective review of medical necessity was against public policy for two reasons. First, it forces patients to choose between following their physician's recommendation for treatment (in which case the patient assumes the risk that the insurer may later deny coverage) and declining to follow the physician's recommendation, possibly foregoing needed treatment. Second, the practice undermines one of the patients' major objectives in being insured: to gain peace of mind that they will not be responsible for the costs of their medical care.

The California Supreme Court concluded that retrospective review of a medical decision in the third-party payer context is not contrary to public policy. In so holding, the court recognized countervailing policy considerations, including the need to preserve alternative health care plans. It noted that the Blue Shield plan, which allows retrospective review, enables the payer to permit the subscriber free selection of a physician and helps maintain relatively low premium rates.

CONCURRENT AND PROSPECTIVE REVIEW

Alternative methods of review include concurrent and prospective review. Under concurrent and prospective review, a third party determines whether care is medically necessary and communicates that decision either before a patient is admitted to a hospital or after admission, but before treatment is actually rendered. While these review methods do not present the patient's dilemma under the retrospective system, a different problem emerges. Here the insurer makes a decision that bears directly on the care rendered to the patient. The burning issue arises as to who may be held responsible for any subsequent harm to a patient who was denied medical treatment based at least in part on the decision of the utilization review organization. Among the candidates for liability are the employer, the patient, the utilization and quality review organizations, the hospital, and the physician. All have separate roles and responsibilities, some or all of which must be taken into consideration in determining liability.[3]

LIABILITY OF UTILIZATION REVIEW ORGANIZATIONS AND PHYSICIANS

Consider first the liability of the utilization review (UR) organization and the physician. The leading case on this issue is *Wickline v. State of California*.[4] In *Wickline*, the payer was the State of California, under its Medi-Cal program. Ms. Wickline was a Medi-Cal patient who had obtained proper authorization for a surgical procedure and ten days of hospitalization. After surgery, complications developed, and Ms. Wickline's physicians sought authorization for an eight-day extension of her stay. Medi-Cal granted only a four-day extension of stay.

Ms. Wickline's physicians discharged her after the four-day extension without appealing Medi-Cal's determination that such a stay would be adequate. After discharge, Ms. Wickline developed medical problems that ultimately resulted in the amputation of her leg above the knee.

Ms. Wickline sued Medi-Cal for wrongfully refusing to approve the requested additional eight days of hospitalization. A jury awarded her $500,000.

Medi-Cal appealed the verdict. The Court of Appeals reversed it, holding that Medi-Cal was not liable for Ms. Wickline's injuries as a matter of law. The court held that the discharge decision is solely the responsibility of the patient's treating physician and that a third-party payer, acting in accordance with appropriate standards of practice, cannot be held legally responsible for subsequent injury to a patient where the discharging physician does not appeal the third-party payer's determination.

While *Wickline* limits a third-party payer's liability if its cost containment program is adequately designed and implemented, it also makes clear that third-party payers may be liable to patients for injuries resulting from inappropriate care under certain circumstances.

The court in *Wickline* made several findings that warrant discussion. First, the court concluded that the decision to discharge a patient is the responsibility of the patient's own treating physician. In *Wickline*, medical expert witnesses for both the plaintiff and the state agreed that the patient's treating physician should decide the course of treatment and determine whether acute care hospitalization is required and for how long. Further, the court said that the patient's physician is in a better position than a Medi-Cal consultant to determine the number of days medically necessary for the required care. The medical experts' agreement was founded on acceptable standards of medical practice as they existed in January 1977. Unless and until medical practice on these issues changes, the court's statement on this issue should provide a reliable guide for third-party payers.

Second, in *Wickline*, no attempt was made by either the attending physicians or the hospital to question the decision or appeal it. The court specifically held that since the patient's treating physicians complied with the judgment of the medical consultant without protest at the time of her discharge, "there can be no viable cause of action against [Medi-Cal] for the consequences of that discharge decision."[5] Thus, the physician carries the burden to persuade the payer's consultants to approve the request. Acquiesence in the payer's determination of what is medically necessary will not shield the physician from liability.[6]

The physician, as underscored in *Wickline*, is charged with the primary obligation of providing the care for the patient. Physicians must be aware that their judgment can be questioned or reviewed by another medical provider, health care insurer, or peer review organization. Accordingly, physicians must document their decisions, clearly laying out the reasons and criteria so that decisions can be reviewed quickly and efficiently. If physicians disagree with the UR organization's decision disapproving of medical treatment or hospitalization, they must seek reconsideration or initiate an appeal, documenting all efforts made in the process.

Third, because the court left open the possiblity of third-party payer liability where there are defects in the design or implementation of cost containment mechanisms, explicit standards for third-party payer performance may be significant. In *Wickline*, Medi-Cal was held to standards set forth in the California Administrative Code. Private third-party payers, not governed by the Administrative Code, must rely on the standards set forth in their agreements with hospitals, physicians, employers, and others. All such agreements should require physicians and hospitals to notify the third-party payer if they disagree with its medical determination. Such a provision is consistent with, and implements, the holding in *Wickline* that the patient's physician is primarily responsible for patient care and is in a better position to determine the medical necessity of that care. If routine processing of the request for care results in an erroneous decision, the physician has a responsibility to object, and the third-party payers should have both an opportunity and a responsibility to review that decision. This protects all parties: the third-party payer has an opportunity to reconsider its initial determination and avoid liability to the patient; the physician (who might well be liable along with the third-party payer for inappropriate care) is protected from liability to the patient; and the patient is protected against receiving inadequate care.

Fourth, the facts in *Wickline* concerning Medi-Cal's review are significant. There, Medi-Cal relied only on the information contained in the form used to request an extension of stay. The Medi-Cal consultant did not review other medical information that would have been available to him from earlier forms in connection with the patient's care. In addition, the Medi-Cal consultant did not initiate telephone calls to the patient's treating physicians. The court tacitly approved these medical procedures. Nevertheless, third-party payers will be better protected by making its review procedures explicit in its agreements with hospitals, physicians, employers, and others. By doing so, providers and practitioners are put on notice that the third-party payer's determination is based only on information supplied in the request submitted and that if further information should be considered it is the responsibility of the practitioners or provider to bring such information to the attention of the third-party payer.

Fifth, although the court did not expressly address the point, it is important to note that the Medi-Cal consultant in *Wickline* was board-certified in general surgery and that the treating physician was a specialist in periperal vascular surgery. The Medi-Cal regulations require that the determination of need for acute care shall be made in accordance with the usual standards of medical practice in the community. It can be argued from the facts and holding in *Wickline* that a third-party payer's consultant should be qualified in

243

the appropriate specialty, but need not be qualified in the subspecialty involved.

EMPLOYER AND HOSPITAL

The employer and the hospital also have significant roles in the utilization review process. The employer has an obligation to educate its employees about the health care organization with which it contracts. The employees should be provided with information about their rights and responsibilities, as well as the procedures and protocols of the system. The employer also has a responsibility to choose an adequate utilization organization. In effect, when the UR organization determines that a particular procedure or treatment plan is not medically necessary, the ultimate decision as to payment remains with the employer. The UR organization will be the employer's expert witness in any related legal action. Therefore, the employer must be sure that the UR organization is competent, professionally recognized, and independent.

Similarly, hospitals must participate in the UR process. Hospitals should refer conflicts between a treating physician or health care provider and the payer's consultant to its own peer review committee. Most hospitals already have such committees in place. Intervention by the hospital review committee at this stage would serve two functions. One function would be to determine whether the hospital concurs with the attending physician's order of the particular care in question and would be willing to defend that physician's position. (This would also provide physicians their own body of experts.) Two, such review assists the hospital in monitoring the performance of physicians and other medical care providers in the institution.

Although hospital staff committee intervention appears to suggest a fairly cumbersome process, it can, in reality, achieve a physician-to-physician consultation within a relatively short period of time. Further, it provides physicians three different perspectives conferring on a problem which is likely to produce a sound medical judgment as to the necessity of medical care. The physician's initial determination could be upheld, modified, or rejected. In cases where the employer is involved, it may be wise to include a mechanism where the employer can overrule the UR organization's recommendation and incur the necessary cost to provide the care for its own, nonmedical reasons.

Communication between treating physicians, UR organizations, patients, and employers at the time the UR decision is being made can go a long way to making intelligent and correct decisions which are both medically necessary and cost-efficient. In advance of that goal, the health care system should provide for physician-to-physician dialogue and an efficient means of gathering and presenting information.

CONCLUSION

Courts have adopted the position that the treating physician is ultimately responsible for the care and treatment of the patient and is the primary candidate for liability. In light of patient needs and the treating physician's access to patient information, the court's direction is warranted. Nevertheless, third-party payers, in designing and implementing cost containment systems involving utilization review mechanisms, are well advised to ensure that their system does not inadvertently or inappropriately usurp primary responsibility for the patient's care and well-being. In assuming patient responsibility, they will also assume legal responsibility for adverse outcomes upon which liability may be assessed.

NOTES

1. While retrospective review has no direct bearing on the care rendered to a patient, the prospect of such a review is likely to influence the physician's judgment. Awareness that medical decisions will be reviewed for cost efficiency has become an element of the environment in which a physician practices and therefore may be taken into account in determining the standard of care in a malpractice action. This subject is beyond the scope of this chapter and has been thoroughly explored in various law review articles. *See*, e.g., Comment, *California Negotiated Health Care: Implications for Malpractice Liability*, 21 San Diego L. Rev. 455 (1984); Schuck, *Malpractice Liability and the Rationing of Care*, 59 Tex. L. Rev. 1421 (1981).

2. 43 Cal. 3d 1, 729 P.2d 267 (1987).

3. Within the Medicare context, peer review organizations (PRO) operate under explicit statutory guideline(s) and receive legal protection for their actions. A PRO is granted immunity from suit as long as it has exercised due care in the performance of its functions. While the private sector has recognized the importance of cost effective health care and has implemented a peer review structure, the law does not yet recognize any qualified or absolute immunity on behalf of such organizations.

4. 192 Cal. App. 3d 1630 (1986).

5. Id at 9.

6. Of course, the physician would not be liable despite his failure to object to the payer's decision if the course of treatment, i.e., withholding care, was reasonable under the circumstances, i.e., not negligent. In addition, in order for persons to be held liable, their negligence must have been the cause of the victim's injury.

Chapter 14

Quality as a Social Issue:
A Journalist's Perspective

Emily Friedman

I received a solicitation a while ago from a magazine entitled *Hippocrates*. As such solicitations go, it was not unusual, except in the pitch it presented. There were questions inscribed on the back of the envelope: "Are left-handed people more susceptible to drugs? What will running do to your knees after 500 miles? Will the right vegetables really help you avoid cancer?" These are intriguing questions, although I am not sure there is such a thing as a right or wrong vegetable. The key question, however, was emblazoned across the front of the envelope. It showed a patient's-eye view of a surgical team, scrubbed and gowned, peering balefully at the reader, waving scalpels. The caption to this threatening scene: "DO THEY KNOW WHAT THEY'RE DOING?"

That question is being asked more and more these days. As health care financing changes, the issues are raised: What is the quality of American health care? How can it be measured? How consistent is it over time? Is it going downhill as health care is reconfigured?

There have been attempts in the past to answer such queries. Quality assurance has been around for a long time, in and out of health care. For example, one approach to quality assurance in musical performance was implicit in a sign spied by Oscar Wilde in a Denver saloon in the last century: "PLEASE DO NOT SHOOT THE PIANO PLAYER; HE IS DOING HIS BEST."

I am not sure we have made all that much progress in quality assurance since those halcyon days of yore. In health care, at least, we have the rather odd spectacle of attorneys serving as the front line of defense in the quality wars. In ten years, however, there will be one million lawyers in the United States. That could lead to so much legal health care quality assurance that those patients

247

who survive the alleged malpractice will die of old age before a judgment is rendered.

Malpractice litigation, as a quality assurance mechanism, has two other problems. One is that it is grievously retroactive. Dead patients may tell no tales, but they also do not benefit much from the settlement. The other is that as the malpractice debate continues unabated, physicians are countersuing attorneys; attorneys are suing each other; medical societies are fighting government; consumer groups are fighting the medical societies; and most of those involved appear to be working at cross-purposes.

Malpractice suits are not likely to provide the final answer in the quality debate. But how can we, trapped in this hall of mirrors--political, social, clinical, and historical--determine what constitutes high quality in health care?

A RELATIVE CONCEPT

First, we should understand that quality is a relative concept, both in terms of what it is and in terms of who says it is what it is. There is no "magic bullet" here--an acceptable definition of quality that everyone will agree on. The situation is similar to that of the unfortunate piano player in Denver: he was at risk because people might not like his selection of tunes, his arrangements, how well he executed them, or his looks. Meanwhile, someone in the audience might have decided to shoot him because the music was boring, or because the beer was warm, or because he was just not having a very good day. In all cases, the review mechanism was a bit arbitrary.

Still, we must try to set some ground rules about health care quality, because without a baseline of some kind, it is very difficult to know what it is we are measuring. More important, without a baseline, we cannot determine if changes in financing and incentives have hurt quality, or helped it, or affected it one way or another.

THE QUALITY OF PROCESS

There are several perspectives from which we might seek to achieve this baseline. One way is to look at the quality of process. This is one of the traditional ways to assess quality. If we counted all the sponges, if all the indicated tests were performed, and if the patient was not left under the X-ray machine too long, then we must have provided good care. Accreditation through the Joint Commission on Accreditation of Healthcare Organizations and approval by third-party payers have long been based on this idea.

The payers--who were more complacent at one time than they are now--assumed that good process meant good outcomes. They figured that the professions were monitoring themselves. They assumed that all doctors were good doctors and all nurses were good nurses and all hospitals were good hospitals. If the process was correct, the operation was a success. Unfortunately, the patient, in some cases, died anyway. But the important thing was that the operation was a success.

But payers' attitudes changed--and quite quickly, given the elephantine pace at which the American health policy process is normally conducted. In 1974, the U.S. House of Representatives' Committee on Ways and Means, by one vote, failed to approve the Kennedy-Mills national health insurance bill. Two years later, Jimmy Carter was elected president, bringing with him Joseph Califano, who, as Secretary of the Department of Health, Education, and Welfare (later, Health and Human Services), put a voice to the growing rumblings about how much health care cost. Health care policy began to shift. From that point on, both public and private payers became far more devoted to containing--and, where possible, cutting --costs than to other issues. Given that all health policy is based on three factors--cost, quality, and access--that relentlessly collide with each other, the popular view among providers was that the ascension of cost was achieved at the price of a lessening of concern about either access or quality.

The health care system was unprepared for this turn of events. It had long followed the thinking of Rene Descartes, who uttered the immortal and fallacious line, "I think, therefore I am." American health care was in the habit of thinking, "I am American health care, and therefore I am great." This attitude was not surprising in a country where providing health care has long been viewed by those who do the providing as an ethical good in and of itself ("I am a doctor, or a nurse, or a hospital, and therefore anything I do is ethically sound").

For a long time, that attitude was a sufficient definition of high quality in health care. But when cost became king, providers suddenly realized that there was no yardstick for quality. They were faced with the grim reality that if all they had to lean on was their contention that whatever they did automatically constituted high quality, they were resting on a slim reed indeed. They had no objective means of documenting their fears that cost cutting and other changes were hurting quality. They did not have the proper tools to do so. They did, however, at least have the sense to ask what all the changes might mean for quality. When the incentives are to provide less care rather than more, what does that mean for patients? When length of stay plummets like a stone, is fat or are muscle and nerve being sliced away? And when payers all jump on the cost-control bandwagon without listening to dissenting voices, who speaks for the patient?

Who indeed? What is worrisome about the suddenness with which values have changed in health care is that hardly anyone did, in fact, ask the patient. For although towers are crumbling and the profession of medicine is being turned on its ear and hospitals are being told that they are outmoded, one of health care's least attractive traditions has held: the patient is too often simply an entity to which other people do things. In the old teaching hospitals, the low-income sick people upon whose bodies research and teaching were conducted were commonly referred to as "clinical material." That attitude has extended in time and scope far beyond the sick poor of yesteryear.

If policymakers and payers, in the process of reconfiguring insurance and delivery systems, had asked the patient what he or she thought of the goings-on, the truth would have been revealed: patients want high-quality, reliable care, and they are far more concerned about that than about costs.[1] A survey of Americans conducted for *Health Management Quarterly* (HMQ) found, for example, that in response to the question, "What do you consider the single most important factor in deciding where to go for medical care?", 50 percent cited "quality of care."[2] Another 25 percent cited "relationship with physician"--that is, a satisfactory trust and power relationship, which is directly related to quality.[2] Another survey found that more than 20 percent of patients switch doctors because they are dissatisfied with the care they receive; and that, in some areas of the country, nearly 40 percent of those surveyed had changed doctors at least once.[3]

In contrast, a relatively meager 14 percent of respondents to the HMQ survey cited cost as the most important factor in choosing providers (see note 2). The groups citing cost most often were black Americans (25 percent) and low-income Americans (32 percent). For many of these people, cost must be a consideration; there is so much health care they cannot afford.

In other words, patients are very concerned about quality. They would prefer not to die of what ails them, and what that survival costs the individual or society is secondary. As Willie said to Joe in the old Bill Mauldin cartoon, "The hell this ain't the most important foxhole in the world; I'm in it!"

Furthermore, patients--and, for that matter, potential patients --are usually not in a position to make clinical judgments. There is more and more talk these days about how patients should take responsibility for their health care decisions and that patients should know how to choose the right provider. We throw television programs, mortality rates, yoga, and broccoli at them and say that if they run into trouble, it is their own fault for being imprudent patients or purchasers.

Although consumerism is an exceedingly powerful and appropriate force in health care, it is possible to carry it too far. If providers and payers are allowed to push off onto the patient major decisions regarding clinical quality, then the patient can be charged with determining what constitutes high or low quality. The providers and payers can then hold themselves blameless for whatever happens --at least until the plaintiff's attorney comes calling.

But people in general, and patients in particular--precisely because they are sick--should not be asked to change professions in mid-fever. They are not clinicians, and they usually cannot make clinical decisions. As Mitchell T. Rabkin, M.D., president of Beth Israel Hospital, Boston, has observed, patients can usually tell the difference between Class A and Class F care; but they aren't too good at detecting all the gradients in-between (see note 1). I smell a rat when people who have, for the most part, been left out of the health care decision-making process are suddenly welcomed into it with open arms and handed a hot potato.

THE QUALITY OF ACCOUNTABILITY

Another form of quality is the quality of accountability (i.e., the question of who is responsible when quality suffers). In other words, who's in charge? There are a number of volunteers for that role these days, some of them very strange bedfellows. Physicians, who have traditionally been quite conservative, are starting to ally themselves with patients and consumer groups on some quality issues --and against a conservative federal administration. The Health Care Financing Administration (HCFA), which helped create the incentives and structures that have led to many of the concerns, is saying that quality is among its top priorities, and that its cost containment efforts have not hurt quality.

Private payers and employers say that quality is a main concern of theirs as well. The growing interest of payers in quality issues does seem appropriate, as it now appears they may be sued for policies that compromise quality in the name of cost. The best known example to date is the *Wickline* case in California, in which a woman sued both her doctor and Medi-Cal (the state Medicaid program), claiming that a premature discharge forced by the program led to the amputation of her leg because of a resulting infection. (See Chapter 13.) On appeal, the court found the state not liable, because the physician went along with the decision. The court further found that the physician, in acquiescing to the Medi-Cal denial of further hospital care, did not act in the patient's best interest. It is likely that there will be similar suits in the future.

In Wisconsin, a Medicaid client who was enrolled in a health maintenance organization, as she was required to do by the state, was refused permission by utilization reviewers to bring her child to an emergency department. The child died, and the mother sued the HMO. The case is still in litigation, but it has already indicated that the chain of accountability--and liability--is beginning to include the payers.

More charitably, private payers and employers--and most public payers as well--know that employees and beneficiaries want the care they receive to be of high or, at least, acceptable quality. Payers and employers also know that if they do not provide such assurance to those whom they are charged with protecting, those people may go elsewhere--if they can. If they have no choice, there is always an available courtroom in which to settle differences of opinion.

Also, public payers are trapped in a maze of conflicting demands. In many rural areas, as well as some urban locales, health care competes directly with the library, fire department, and schools for scarce resources. A majority of states are facing financial difficulties. They have tough choices to make, and Medicaid remains one of the top two or three budget items in every state. On the federal level, there are questions of "macro-allocation," or deciding between B-1 bombers and bassinets.

Health care policy is conducted on the grand scale by government, as it must be. And some insensitivity inevitably results from that. As a health policy analyst named Harry S. Mustard observed about hit-and-miss government regulation of meat processing plants in the early twentieth century, "The state as a whole did not smell the odor of a local slaughterhouse."[4]

However, there is a difference between the unavoidable insensitivity of regulation and ignoring the basic responsibility of government as an agent of society. Government is supposed to implement the will of the people, when it can figure out what that will is. And government should know that people want to trust their health care providers--that people expect that even if the state does not smell the slaughterhouse, it will listen to those who do. It is therefore troublesome that HCFA was in no hurry in 1985-1986 to initiate quality review of the HMOs in which the better part of a million Medicare beneficiaries had signed up. Congress finally had to mandate that something be done. In the meantime, the nation was treated to the sad affair of International Medical Centers (IMC) in Florida.

IMC was an HMO with a questionable record in a number of areas. Nevertheless, it had signed up the largest number of Medicare beneficiaries of any HMO in the country. Subscribers and contractors complained in growing numbers about abuses, but the federal government failed to respond. This may or may not have been connected to the fact that IMC had hired a small herd of former federal officials. After a year's delay, the president of IMC was indicted on racketeering charges, and the organization was turned over to the state of Florida. Even the federal government finally cancelled its Medicare contract with IMC--months after the barn door had been left wide open. The HMO was eventually sold to the Humana health care chain.

Another interesting example of government's attitude toward quality assurance was the controversy over Paracelsus Healthcare, a proprietary firm in California that featured extraordinary alleged billing practices, such as charging the government for country club fees. The Department of Health and Human Services decided that

Paracelsus should pay $4.45 million to the department--and provide $100,000 in free care to the medically indigent residents of southern California. Given that Paracelsus was first called on the carpet for allegedly shoddy practices, it is unsettling that part of its punishment was to offer those shoddy services to the poor. Indeed, one can discern in this byzantine settlement an ironic illustration of the interaction of cost, quality, and access.

The Failure of Self-Policing

However, before providers gloat about the clumsiness of some payers in the arena of accountability, they should realize that third-party payers--public and private alike--intervened because providers had not distinguished themselves in terms of self-policing. No entity that has a choice will step into the line of accountability, and thus of potential legal liability, unless it perceives that no one is minding the store. Providers must understand that, other considerations aside, one reason there is so much malpractice litigation is that there is a great deal of malpractice.

Paul Ellwood, M.D., chairman of Interstudy, uttered a great truth when he said, "Physicians came to be health care leaders because of their ability to resist change."[5] That was true when it came to quality. They, and the hospitals in which they worked, fed the conspiracy of silence that enshrouded health care quality. The operation was a success. The patient died. The lawyer sued.

Fewer Days

Another aspect of accountability is the diminishing length of time for which any one provider is responsible for a patient. Hospital length of stay for patients overall in late 1987 was down to approximately 6.6 days; Medicare length of stay was approximately 8.8 days. Less care is provided in the inpatient setting; more is provided in the physician's office, the outpatient department, the nursing home, and the home itself. Even HMOs appear to push you out the door as soon as possible. For an extended illness, there is often little central coordination. No one may be accountable for the patient over the entire period of the illness. The patient who was handed the hot potato of determining what good care is has now become a hot potato himself.

This ping-ponging does not breed the trust and confidence that are requisite components of high-quality health care. And patients can become suspicious about it. Claude Lewis, a *Philadelphia Inquirer* columnist, wrote in that paper on January 25, 1986, that when he developed eye trouble, he was bounced around among an HMO, a primary care physician, an answering service, and a computer. The delay could have been tragic, given that he is diabetic. "It seems unusual," he wrote, "for anyone to awaken with severe pain and redness after going to bed feeling completely normal. Yet the system is such that patient input is of little or no consequence.... It seems to me that emergency rooms, hospitals, doctors, and the federal government, with its DRGs, are hampering good health. For good health, in my view, is not merely the absence of illness, but the presence of confidence in the medical system that is supposed to provide adequate care."[6]

Who is accountable? This will be the payers' department exclusively if providers do not take more responsibility for both their actions and their inaction--and those of their peers. And the payers' agenda may be far different than that of those who provide care.

THE QUALITY OF QUANTITY

The crux of the matter may be yet another kind of quality: the quality of quantity and our inability to tell the one from the other. In this land of plenty, we have traditionally viewed quality and quantity as interchangeable. Bigger is better. Who scores the most points? What costs the most? Whose car is biggest?

This value, long one of the wellsprings of American culture, has started to change. Fat, which was fashionable when it was rare, is replaced by lean. Less is more, the architects say. Small is beautiful. We shrink the scope of things to a more personal level, coming up with such creations as the "personal business copier," an apparent contradiction in terms.

In health care, of course, quantity *was* quality. We rewarded quantity. We applauded the sort of "Star Trek" mentality that advocated going to new worlds, meeting new people, and trying new things. We were supposed to "go for it," clinically speaking. Even in health care, we were captives of the idea of manifest destiny, driven by our need to know.

That manifest curiosity produced an ever-increasing quantity of effort, and we came to accept quantity and quality as interchangeable in health care. We began to make a science of the art of medicine, tying it to hematocrit and blood pressure levels, T4s, and CT and MRI readings. Physicians and nurses became more and more expert at using sophisticated quantitative tools to measure, and thereby improve, health care. And we were perfectly happy with the quantification of care. As long as the numbers were used to justify the continued expansion of the health care system, there were few complaints.

However, as the great American Zen philosopher, Yogi Berra, has noted, "You can observe a lot just by watching." And there were elves about. They took the methodologies and ideas that were guiding the clinical laboratory and the radiology department and started using them, not to diagnose the individual patient, but to diagnose the process of health care itself. That led to a fundamental change in values, a root-shaking re-evaluation of the quality of quantity.

What Have We Learned?

We have learned from the work of John Wennberg, M.D., of the Department of Community and Family Medicine at Dartmouth Medical School, and his fellow researchers that patients undergo many surgical and medical procedures at strikingly different rates, even when they live very near each other.[7] It seems that when there is not consensus on how to treat a condition, physicians can be quite inconsistent in how they go about treating it. In some cases, several different approaches are equally appropriate. In other cases, overtreatment may well be occurring. In yet other situations, undercare may be taking place.

Dedicated physicians are working to resolve the riddle of practice pattern variation and to rationalize those variations. The Maine Medical Assessment Project and similar efforts in Maryland are using practice pattern variations to develop clinical consensus: to understand why doctors make the decisions they do, and to set parameters by which questionable patterns of care can be monitored. (See Chapter 8.)

Another procedure has passed from the realm of possible over-occurrence into the stratosphere of inappropriate care: cesarean section. Fifteen years ago, the U.S. rate was 6.5 percent of all deliveries; today, it is almost 25 percent.[8] In some areas, it is much higher. In metropolitan Miami, for example, among privately insured women, the rate is an eye-catching 42 percent.[9] Furthermore, a study in New York City of 65,000 deliveries found that women being treated by private physicians ran a much higher chance of cesarean section than women treated by house staff or attending physicians in public hospitals.[10] This finding gives every impression of an economic motive, regardless of pious explanations about malpractice and patient choice.

Health services research has raised other questions. There are several procedures, including coronary artery bypass grafts, heart transplants, and several more common operations, for which it has been demonstrated that the greater the number performed in a hospital, the better the outcome.[11] (See Chapter 2.) Evaluations based on such findings led the Veterans Administration to close some of its cardiac surgery units, which were experiencing relatively poor outcomes. Researchers are now asking if this relationship of volume and mortality is true of the individual doctor who performs the procedure.

Yet providers still scramble to start or retain low-volume services that are likely to have, or do have, subpar outcomes because they might offer some marginal marketing advantage. For instance, a recent study reported a fifteen per cent mortality rate for cardiac catheterizations in one California hospital. This rate is far in excess of average mortality for this procedure.[12] It does not take sophisticated analysis to recognize that something is probably quite wrong at that facility.

The quality/quantity interface works both ways. Providers have tended to think that a reduction of the amount of care automatically threatened quality. But quality can also be compromised by the provision of too much care; health services can be quite dangerous, and should not be provided for reasons of economics or ego.

The quality of quantity must be judged in two other ways. One is that we tend to concentrate on the life-and-death procedure --the transplant, the artificial organ. These exotic procedures represent only a tiny fraction of health care encounters, however. More commonly, patients seek treatment for sinusitis, a minor fever, or bunions. We tend to discount the importance of examining such encounters in terms of their frequency or appropriateness, because there is no harm done, we say, if we do a little too much here or there. But when it's your foxhole, you take it all seriously. As Bill Walton, the great basketball player who has undergone many surgical procedures, observed, "I learned a long time ago that minor surgery is when they are doing it to somebody else."

When Do We Stop?

The other aspect of the quality of quantity is that the health care system has yet to learn when to stop. It is absurd that too often physicians and hospitals force care on people who no longer want it and who can no longer benefit from it, when at the same time there is massive payer pressure on providers to offer less care.

One of the most poignant interviews in this regard was that conducted with William Bartling, a terminally ill Californian, who was suing the hospital that had placed him in an intensive care unit and was forcing treatment on him when he wanted to be allowed to die.[13] He had been attached to a ventilator against his will. He was asked, "Do you want to die, Bill?" He responded no, he did not want to die. He was then asked, "Do you want to be on this ventilator?" He responded no, he did not want to be. He was then asked, "Do you understand that if we disconnect the ventilator, you will die?" He nodded yes, he understood that. Incredibly, the judge ruled that this indicated that he was ambivalent and therefore should stay on the ventilator! William Bartling died before the case was settled, although his estate and family won it shortly afterward. What the judge did not understand was that people like Mr. Bartling will trade the quantity of a life for its quality. It is a lesson that the guardians of such patients learn too rarely--and often too late.

Similarly, in Chicago in 1986, a seven-month-old child named Meghann LaRocco was subjected to four liver transplants. The third liver came from a burn victim and the odds were overwhelming that it would not "take," which it did not. The child's father had announced publicly that he would stop at three procedures. But when the third liver began to fail, he approved a fourth transplant. He told an interviewer that he did not want to be wondering, a week later, if there was something more he could have done for his child, but did not. Meghann has survived it all, so far. But was this a good use of resources? There are dozens of children waiting for donor livers, and dozens who die for lack of them--or for lack of money to pay for them.

Albert Einstein said, "Perfection of means and confusion of goals characterize the age." David Willis, editor of the *Milbank Quarterly*, has said that our ability to create technology has outstripped our ability to internalize its implications. Now that the secrets of what Dr. John Wennberg calls the "black box" of medicine are starting to be revealed, we must learn to use the information wisely--not to defend overcare or undercare, not to prop up faulty policy decisions, not to torment patients at the end of their lives, not to underwrite corporate profits or professional ego. We must divorce quality and quantity and remarry them in a more sensible union.

THE QUALITY OF CARING

That moves the discussion to the quality of caring. This is different from the technical quality of care. It is also different from the quality of curing, with which we are obsessed--which is why Mr. Bartling had such a rough time.

The quality of caring is under assault, and nowhere so much as in nursing. A nursing shortage has cropped up again, with the American Hospital Association reporting a 1986 hospital nursing vacancy rate of 13.6 percent--double the 1985 rate of 6.3 percent. A survey by the American Organization of Nurse Executives found that 83 percent of U.S. hospitals had vacancies.

Why are people leaving nursing, or at least hospital nursing? One major reason is that they feel they are being denied the right to do their jobs; that is, to provide clinically appropriate, humane, sensitive care. With all the cutbacks in FTEs and shorter lengths of stay, who has the time to visit with Mrs. Smith and admire the baby? Who can chat with Mr. Jones and look at the picture of the new grandchild? Can enough time be freed to hold Charlie's hand as he slips quietly from this world, or should he be left to die alone? These are the kinds of decisions one would expect battlefield medics to have to make, not professionals in a $500 billion health care economy. A decline in the quality of caring affects patient perceptions as well. A Voluntary Hospitals of America study found that one of two key factors influencing patient impressions of the quality

259

of care is "caring attitudes of hospital employees."[14] The other is medical staff qualifications.

Yet even prestigious patients can encounter problems in this regard. *Newsweek* senior editor Meg Greenfield, in a memorable 1986 article, described her experience in what she termed "the land of hospital."[15] She described it as: "A nation--a universe, really, of its own, within which one quickly and progressively sinks into the role of patient, analogous in the way it transforms your personality and gnaws at both your assurance and sense of self to being a tourist in an unfathomable, dangerous land." And how did the tourist guides treat her? She describes "the distinctive, essential hospital experience of our times" as "a maddening combination of individual excellence and systemic incompetence, the one tirelessly and heroically saving life and limb, the other forever putting both at mindless risk."

Another aspect of the quality of caring has to do with an all-too-familiar type of patient, described by Paul Ruskin, M.D., as follows: "A white female who appears her reported age. She neither speaks nor comprehends the spoken word. Sometimes she babbles incoherently for hours on end. She is disoriented about person, place, and time. She does, however, seem to recognize her own name. I have worked with her for the past six months, but she does not recognize me."[16] Ruskin pointed out that the patient was virtually helpless; had to be fed, clothed, and bathed by others; and was incontinent to boot. He asked a group of graduate nurses how they would feel about dealing with such a case. They responded with words like "frustrated," "hopeless," "depressed," and "annoyed." Ruskin was describing his six-month-old daughter.

We have long have been wed to the curative and are hesitant to think in terms of the incurable. However, neither nursing, medicine, nor any other health care profession comes with a guarantee that its members will be called upon only to practice what Ronald Anderson, M.D., director of Parkland Memorial Hospital in Dallas, describes as "resurrection medicine." One takes a vow, as a caregiver, to do no harm and to try to give comfort. Yet we have somehow overlooked that in favor of doing everything possible to heal a patient with acute illness, while we often do little when confronted by chronic illness. We should not define provider success solely in terms of complete cure in acute illness, and we certainly cannot cling to such a definition in the future.

Patients at the extremes--the very old, the very sick, the dying--are the most intractable, but they also are the neediest, the loneliest, the most responsive to caring. Curing and caring are both important; but they are different. Sometimes the most uncaring thing we can do is demand too much from patients who cannot respond. We should not make people feel that they are failures because they cannot get well.

Caring and quality are directly related in another way. Consider this frightening and critically important malpractice case: A young woman named Susan von Stetina was badly hurt in an auto accident.[17] She was admitted, with severe head injuries, to an overflowing ICU that was insufficiently staffed. She suffered brain damage during the night and lapsed into an irreversible coma. Her family won its malpractice suit against the hospital in part because of evidence as to who was in the ICU that night. Among the clientele was a person declared brain dead a few hours later, and two others scheduled to be voluntarily discharged from the hospital the next morning. Yet they absorbed the time of the nursing staff, and Susan von Stetina slipped away.

It is no coincidence that the editorial accompanying the report of this case in the *Journal of the American Medical Association* was written by William Knaus, M.D., of George Washington University Medical Center.[18] (See Chapter 4.) He and his colleagues found, in a study of survival rates in ICUs in major medical centers, that a patient's chances of survival may well be directly tied to the amount of autonomy the ICU nurses have.[19] In an eerie reflection of the von Stetina tragedy, they found that hospitals with very good ICU survival rates have extremely positive nurse-physician relationships. In at least one institution, the charge nurse had the right, autonomously, to cancel elective surgery if she did not believe there was sufficient nursing staff to ensure good post-operative care.

The concept of teamwork is not simply a "rah-rah" inspirational mechanism. Things tend to go more smoothly when people work well together. In the contemporary hospital, with staff divided by computers, specialization, overwork, and turf battles, the concept of teamwork needs to be reborn; caregivers need to know and care about each other so that they can know and care about their patients.

Teamwork can and should, in fact, go even deeper. In 1984, a young physician wrote about what it is like to be a patient facing a potentially fatal disease. Describing being prepared for a biopsy

261

by his own colleagues, he observed, "All the people I'd seen...I'd worked with on major cases. I had known their level of competence. Yet, even though it turned out that my surgery was so minor I probably could have done it myself, I had been terrified. I later thought of how it is with sick patients who must face surgery alone, among strangers whose competence and kindness have yet to be proved."[20]

THE QUALITY OF QUALITY ASSURANCE

The jury is still out in terms of the quality of quality assurance. It is clear that some of those in power, in both the public and private sectors, would prefer that we take their word that quality is holding its own, without other evidence. This is what I call the "George Brett Rule of Quality Assurance." Jim Frey, at the time the manager of the Kansas City Royals, was once asked what batting advice he gave to George Brett, the team's premier hitter. Frey replied quietly, "I tell him, 'Attaway to hit, George!'"

Quality assurance cannot be left to this sort of blind faith and inattention. Nor can Peer Review Organizations do it alone. (See Chapters 5, 6, and 9.) Despite the excellence of many PROs, and a clear commitment to quality on the part of many of them, I have yet to see the agency that can successfully serve two masters. In the 1970s, Congress created Health Systems Agencies, which were charged with serving both the cause of planning and the cause of cost containment. They often ended up serving neither, because the two sets of goals were often incompatible.

PROs, whatever their charge, are still paid by a financing agency that seeks to pay as little as possible for the care it is required to purchase. This will make life very difficult for the PROs, and I am not sure all of them will be able to surmount the essential contradiction of their situation.

Payers, as a group, face the same conflicts, whether they think quality is suffering, is being enhanced, or neither. If ensuring quality is going to cost them money, they, too, face inherent conflicts. There is some hope in terms of independent agencies, especially the Joint Commission on Accreditation of Healthcare Organizations, which has announced its intention to base accreditation, in part, on outcomes rather than solely on process and on quantitative measures rather than guesswork. (See Chapters 1 and 2.)

But in the end, quality assurance must start with those who are most qualified to define quality. It must start with the providers--hospitals, their trustees, physicians, nurses, and probably social workers and patient advocates as well. They all must serve as the conscience of the system.

In terms of the varieties of quality described in this chapter, who else can guard them? Who else can link (and unlink, when necessary) process with outcome and know what the proper balance is? Who else should be accountable, other than those on whose hands the blood will or will not spill? Who else can unburden us of the myth of quality as quantity, and reforge their relation to each other in keeping with the new realities of research and experience? And who else need concern themselves with the caring aspects of quality--the need to care when cure is not possible, and to respect patients because of the covenant by which they have placed their very lives in the hands of others? If health care providers do not take up quality as a personal cause--not for reasons of marketing advantage, enhancing reimbursement, avoiding malpractice litigation, or professional self-aggrandizement, but because it is an inherent part of the compact they made with society--then all the software, regulations, and consultants in the world will not protect patients, nor those who provide care to them, from a bleak and threatening future.

THE QUALITY OF MERCY

Speaking of protection, there is one more type of quality: the quality of mercy. What has been forgotten, in the debate over cost and quality, is the third part of the equation: access.

While we quibble over whether an injection was given well, we ignore the 35 million or so Americans who lack either public or private health insurance, and who must beg for crumbs at the door.[21] This is the ultimate rationing issue, one of far greater scope than questions of reducing certain kinds of ancillary testing or marginal surgery.

Today, one child receives four liver transplants in a nation with an infant mortality rate of 10.6 children per 1,000--worst in the developed world, despite the fact that we spend more on health care per capita than any other nation.[22] As many as 40 percent of all children aged one to four have not been immunized against measles, rubella, or polio, and the number of cases of measles is doubling annually. Tuberculosis is making a comeback. Our maternal mortality rate for black women is worse than the rates in Singapore and Costa Rica.

The American Cancer Society reports that low-income Americans die of the same cancers, contracted at the same time as those afflicting other Americans, at a rate 10 to 15 percent higher, apparently because they do not get into the health care system in time for care to do them any good.[23] Half of elderly black women live below the poverty line, spending 16 percent of what income they have on out-of-pocket health care expenses. Our streets are strewn with between 250 thousand and 3 million homeless people. Many of these are mentally ill. We discharged them from institutions to the streets, saying that they are not harmful to us. But this turn of events has been harmful to them.

The number of Americans with private health insurance is dropping.[24] Medicaid covers fewer than half of those living below the federal poverty line.[25] Insurers are working overtime to jettison individuals at high risk of contracting acquired immune deficiency syndrome.

There will be other diseases--Huntington's chorea, diabetes, and, in time, cancer--for which we will be able to track people's predisposition at birth. In fact, we may soon have the technical capability to eliminate almost anyone who needs health insurance from the ranks of the insured.

Yet we speak, in hushed tones, of rationing--as though it were not already taking place. We should speak of something else instead. We should speak of *reallocation* of health care resources--of the need to turn away from economic incentives toward clinical incentives, to take what we waste and spend it on those who are being denied. We spend millions of dollars every year on systems designed to keep people from getting health care, through eligibility determinations, screens, and utilization review, driven more by economics than by concerns over appropriateness and application of other criteria. With all this money redirected, we might well have enough money to care for the excluded vulnerable, if we are willing to change.

One cannot discuss quality without discussing the quality of mercy--the ethical value and values of a nation and a health care system that consistently exclude many of the most needy, helpless, and frail. There is no high quality in overtreating a paying patient while children go blind from untreated measles elsewhere in town. There is no morality in implementing major changes in financing on the basis of ideological theory, a lick, and a promise, and then refusing to acknowledge that 15 percent of the population is cascading through the cracks that those changes have widened. Until the door is opened to these people, we are all responsible for what happens to them and to the quality of their care. For the lowest quality health care of all is that which is denied in the face of documented need.

WHAT VERSUS WHOM

Gerald Weissmann, M.D., a professor of medicine at New York University and an internist at Bellevue, has given us perhaps the best description of the sociology of access, cost, and quality--of how the social contract intermeshes with what makes health care tick. He was musing about the new tower building into which Bellevue moved in 1975, and about the oddity of treating society's outcasts in such fancy surroundings.

The infective insults of streptococci and tuberculosis are abetted by poverty, dirt, and urban crowding--what the young leftists of the 1970s called 'disease of oppression.' And since there is little evidence that these social imperfections have been ameliorated, newer diseases of the underclass have begun to replace the old.... We now find our wards filled with cases of AIDS, 'brown heroin kidney,' 'gay bowel,' oral chancres, gonococcal arthritis, the hepatitis of drug abuse or pederasty, the endocarditis relayed by infected needles, and the acute respiratory distress that follows a jet of flaming cocaine....

On the quiet corporate floors of the new hospital tower, the professional middle class (students, house officers, attending physicians) sorts out the ranks of those wounded in our social wars. The mugged, maimed, drugged, and infected are victims of epidemics as virulent as those that filled the gracious loggias [of the old Bellevue] of 1908. The high-rise columns and modular panels of corporate architecture now house the losers of the new urban scrimmages, for whom there is no place in the similar towers of Wall Street or midtown. In both the old Bellevue and the new--and for this reason there is perhaps no more engaging hospital in which to work--we have been able to appreciate not only *what* happens in disease, but also to *whom*.[26]

That is the endpoint of all quality determination. It is not what the numbers say, nor how nice the halls look, not the income or insurance status of the patient; it is to whom the bad things can happen. And the answer to that is, to all of us. We are all potential patients.

What is quality? William Guy, the former head of Blue Cross of California and former commissioner of Medi-Cal, was once asked what quality was. He responded, "What is quality? What *I* do is quality; what *you* do is schlock." That is one way to define quality, and one that could be said to fit right into a competitive market framework.

But the magazine solicitation described at the opening of this chapter asked a more absolute question. It asked whether health care providers know what they are doing. The Greek scholar after whom the magazine is named told health care professionals to ask themselves that question, and suggested they start first by seeing to it that they did no harm. Buddha augmented that idea, in his last words on earth, by counseling his followers, "Do your best."

Taken together, these thoughts constitute a more useful definition of high quality. Remember that it is not *what*, but *whom*. Do no harm. Do your best. Go beyond the philosophical appeal of these concepts and learn what research, experience, courage, and insight can teach us about what they really mean. It is, to be sure, an act of self-defense on the part of providers; but, in the process of wrestling with the issue of quality and coming to peace with definitions and processes we all can live with, providers will be acting in the defense of us all.

NOTES

1. E. Friedman, "What Do Consumers Really Want?", *Healthcare Forum*, 29(May-June 1986): 19.

2. "HMO Survey: A Mandate for High-Quality Care," *Health Management Quarterly*, (Fourth Quarter 1986): 3.

3. "Study Looks at Doctor Switching," *Blue Cross and Blue Shield Media Digest*, 7(Feb. 17, 1987).

4. O. Anderson, *Health Services in the United States* (Ann Arbor, MI: Health Administration Press, 1985).

5. P. Ellwood, presentation at American Hospital Association Trustee Forum, June 12, 1986.

6. C. Lewis, "Beginning to Question Health Care Systems," *Philadelphia Inquirer*, January 25, 1986.

7. E. Friedman, "Practice Variations: Where Will the Push to Fall in Line End?", *Medical World News*, 27(January 27, 1986): 51.

8. E. Friedman, "Looking Ahead: Cesarean Section," *Health Business*, 11(September 19, 1986): 3T.

9. P. Shiono et al., "Recent Rends in Cesarean Birth and Trial of Labor Rates in the United States," *Journal of the American Medical Association*, 257(January 23/30, 1987): 494. See also: N. Gleicher, "Cesarean Section Rates in the United States," *Journal of the American Medical Association*, 252(December 21, 1984): 3273.

10. H. De Regt et al., "Relation of Private or Clinic Care to the Cesarean Birth Rate," *New England Journal of Medicine*, 315(September 4, 1986): 619.

11. E. Friedman, "Payers Act on Volume/Mortality Findings," *Health Business*, 1(December 19, 1986): 3T.

12. H. Luft, "Evaluating Individual Hospital Quality Through Outcome Statistics," *Journal of the American Medical Association*, 255(May 23/30, 1986): 2780.

13. G. Annas, "Prisoner in the ICU: The Tragedy of William Bartling," in *Making Choices: Ethics Issues for Health Care Practitioners*, ed. E. Friedman (Chicago: American Hospital Publishing, Inc., 1986).

14. "Consumers Cite Attributes of Hospital Quality," *Blue Cross and Blue Shield Media Digest*, 9(March 2, 1987).

15. M. Greenfield, "The Land of Hospital," *Newsweek*, June 30, 1986.

16. P. Ruskin, "Aging and Caring," *Journal of the American Medical Association*, 250(Nov. 11, 1983): 2440.

17. H.T. Engelhardt, "Intensive Care Units, Scarce Resources, and Conflicting Principles of Justice," *Journal of the American Medical Association*, 255(March 7, 1986): 1159.

18. W. Knaus, "Rationing, Justice, and the American Physician," *Journal of the American Medical Association*, 255(March 7, 1986): 1176.

19. W. Knaus et al., "An Evaluation of Outcome From Intensive Care in Major Medical Centers," *Annals of Internal Medicine*, 104(March 1986): 410.

20. S. Frank, "Lessons," *Journal of the American Medical Association*, 252(October 19, 1984): 2014.

21. E. Friedman, *Care of the Medically Indigent* (Chicago: American Society for Hospital Planning and Marketing, American Hospital Association, 1986).

22. E. Friedman, "The Health Lifeline: Out of the Reach of Women and Children?", *Hospitals*, 60(October 20, 1986): 46. See also: "U.S. Infant Mortality Rate Dropped in 1984," *Medicine & Health*, 41(April 6, 1987): 2.

23. *Cancer in the Economically Disadvantaged: A Special Report* (New York City: American Cancer Society, 1986).

24. *Source Book of Health Insurance Data: 1986 Update* (Washington, DC: Health Insurance Association of America, 1986).

25. E. Friedman, "Medicaid's Overload Sparks a Crisis," *Hospitals* 61(January 20, 1987): 50.

26. E. Friedman, *Is Counting the Dead Enough?* (New York City: United Hospital Fund, 1986).

27. G. Weissman, "Bellevue: Form Follows Function," in *The Woods Hole Cantata*, G. Weissman (Boston: Houghton Mifflin, 1985).